Our Journey Beyond Sunset Boulevard - Evidence-based Analysis of Tumor-Targeted Gene- and Immuno-Therapies Shine a Critical Spotlight on "True" Long-Term Cancer-Free Survival

Authored by
Erlinda M. Gordon and Frederick L. Hall

Published in London, United Kingdom

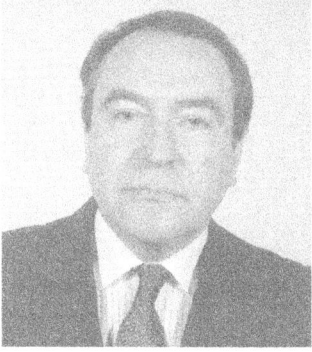

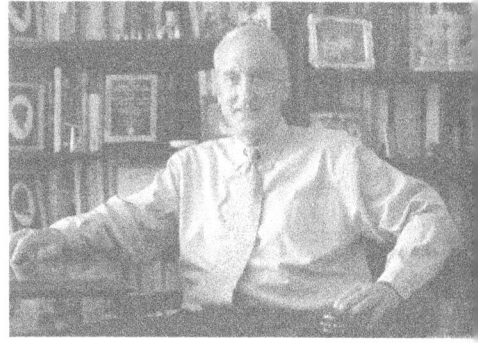

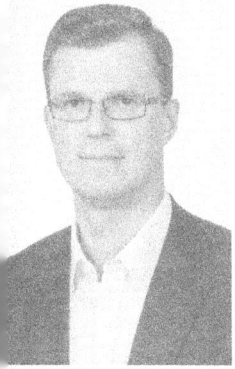

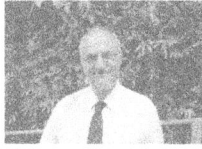

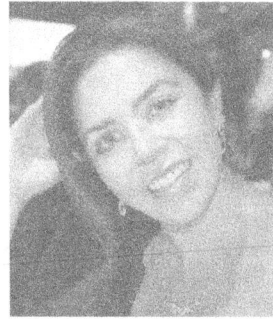

Supporting open minds since 2005

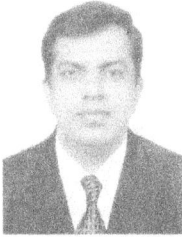

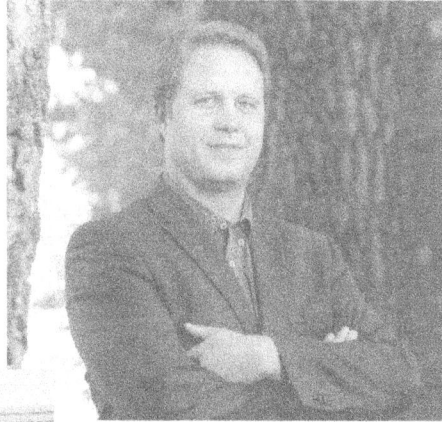

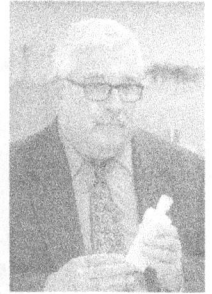

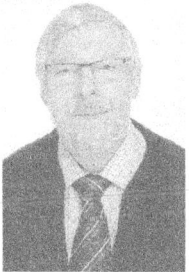

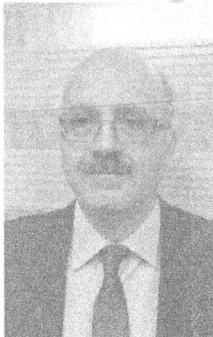

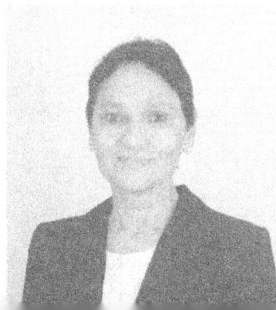

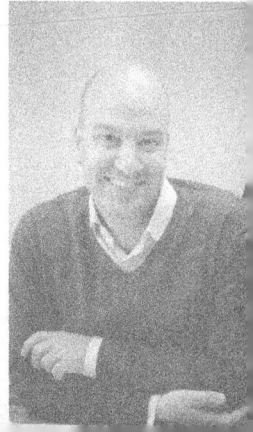

Our Journey Beyond Sunset Boulevard - Evidence-based Analysis of Tumor-Targeted Gene- and Immuno-Therapies Shine a Critical Spotlight on "True" Long-Term Cancer-Free Survival
http://dx.doi.org/10.5772/intechopen.95307
Authored by Erlinda M. Gordon and Frederick L. Hall

Contributors
Erlinda M. Gordon and Frederick L. Hall

Notice
Statements and opinions expressed in the chapters are these of the individual contributors and not necessarily those of the editors or publisher. No responsibility is accepted for the accuracy of information contained in the published chapters. The publisher assumes no responsibility for any damage or injury to persons or property arising out of the use of any materials, instructions, methods or ideas contained in the book.

First published in London, United Kingdom, 2021 by IntechOpen
IntechOpen is the global imprint of INTECHOPEN LIMITED, registered in England and Wales, registration number: 11086078, 5 Princes Gate Court, London, SW7 2QJ, United Kingdom
Printed in Croatia

British Library Cataloguing-in-Publication Data
A catalogue record for this book is available from the British Library

Additional hard and PDF copies can be obtained from orders@intechopen.com

Our Journey Beyond Sunset Boulevard - Evidence-based Analysis of Tumor-Targeted Gene- and Immuno-Therapies Shine a Critical Spotlight on "True" Long-Term Cancer-Free Survival
Authored by Erlinda M. Gordon and Frederick L. Hall
p. cm.
Print ISBN 978-1-83969-415-8
Online ISBN 978-1-83969-416-5
eBook (PDF) ISBN 978-1-83969-417-2

We are IntechOpen,
the world's leading publisher of
Open Access books
Built by scientists, for scientists

5,300+
Open access books available

129,000+
International authors and editors

155M+
Downloads

156
Countries delivered to

Our authors are among the

Top 1%
most cited scientists

12.2%
Contributors from top 500 universities

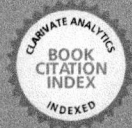

Interested in publishing with us?
Contact book.department@intechopen.com

Numbers displayed above are based on latest data collected.
For more information visit www.intechopen.com

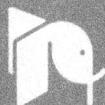

Meet the authors

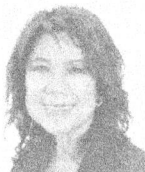

Dr. Erlinda M. Gordon, MD, is a Pediatric Hematologist-Oncologist with extensive experience in the field of gene transfer/gene therapy, specifically in the development of the first and, so far, only, targeted gene vector that has been validated in the clinic. Dr. Gordon served as the Gene Therapy Sponsor and FDA liaison for five US-based Phase I/II clinical trials for pancreatic cancer, sarcoma, and breast cancer and three Philippines-based Phase 1/2 studies for all solid tumors. During her eleven-year term as Chief Medical Officer of Epeius Biotechnologies Corp., DeltaRex-G (formerly Rexin-G) gained US FDA Fast Track status for pancreatic cancer, Orphan Drug designation for pancreatic cancer, osteosarcoma, and soft tissue sarcoma, and accelerated approval for all solid malignancies in the Philippines. Dr. Gordon is the Founder and President of the Aveni Foundation, and under her supervision, DeltaRex-G gained Expanded Access for DeltaRex-G in 2019 and Emergency Use Authorization for COVID-19 in 2020. Dr. Gordon served as Associate Professor of Pediatrics, USC Keck School of Medicine/Children's Hospital of Los Angeles, California, from 1989 to 2013. Dr. Gordon recieved an Award for Excellence in Biotechnology from the Los Angeles City Mayor in 2005 and the Thomas Award for Excellence in Biomedical Research in 2016.

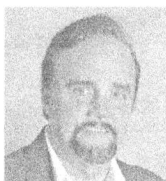

Dr. Frederick L. Hall, Ph.D., is an American scientist whose work in chemical carcinogenesis and molecular cybernetics established the biochemistries and molecular genetics of "Stem Cell Competence" governing the animal cell division cycle. His research laboratory at CHLA discovered/cloned or helped characterize the human EGFr-associated (HERA) Map kinase signaling pathway and the cyclin-dependent kinase pathway in cancer. His pioneering work with Dr. Erlinda M. Gordon, MD, developed DeltaRex-G (formerly Rexin-G) from bench to bedside, establishing Cyclin G1 blockade (dnG1, silver bullet) as a singular, pivotal, and strategic locus for applied/targeted cancer gene therapy. Dr. Hall served progressively as Director of Research in the departments of orthopedic, cardiothoracic, and colorectal cancer surgeries at the USC Keck School of Medicine; former President, CEO, and CSO of Epeius Biotechnologies; acting CSO of the Aveni Foundation rescue mission; current partner in Counterpoint Biomedica and Delta NextGene supportive biotechnology firms. Dr. Hall received the Smith Award for Excellence in Biomedical Research in 1995.

Contents

Preface

The purpose of this book is to convey the hard-fought, hard-won interdisciplinary advances in tumor targeting, cellular cybernetics, oncogene science, and metastatic cancer control achieved with the clinical development of **DeltaRex-G**-*the first proactive tumor-hunting/tumor-killing biomedicine of this kind in history*-**to a layman audience**, including cancer patients, medical students, researchers, and future practitioners in the emerging field of precision-guided gene-based medicine. The historic documentation of physiological tumor surveillance, metastatic cancer eradication, and long-term survival benefits demonstrated in the crucible of clinical oncology, evaluated analytically the context of chemotherapy-resistant cancers, led the US FDA to restore **DeltaRex-G** (formerly Rexin-G) to the original inventors and the cancer clinic with "Expanded Access" in 2019, empowered by the "Right-to-Try" legislation, now US law.

The format of the discourse is decidedly educational (allegorical, illustrative, and picturesque), realizing that a cancer patient's "Right-to-Try" eligible experimental therapies in the United States is guided by the ethical principles of "informed consent," which demands a high level of truthfulness in both logic and diction, faithful adherence to governing regulatory covenants, and reliable quantification in terms of evidence-based claims of tumor targeting, general drug safety, and predictable clinical efficacy. Herein, the authors utilize the revealing powers of allegory and classic literature, adding shared iconic cinematic experiences of postmodernism, at times, to educate, inform, and convey the **hard-core science**; that is, the fundamental *biochemistries, biophysics, molecular biology, cancer genetics, stem cell biology, regulatory biology, synthetic virology, tumor immunology, clinical oncology, bio-pharmacology, histopathology, and gene-based therapy* embodied within the **"smart"** therapeutic nanoparticle now called **DeltaRex-G**.

The book is organized into seven sections, each designed to engage the layman (postmodern, post-Enlightenment reader) conceptually, and to enable the reader to visually and intuitively approach biomedically complex, often confusing, rapidly evolving, inscrutable, and/or esoteric cancer biology with relative ease. The book accomplishes this with the assistance of a compassionate (no-nonsense) narrator, several utilitarian "characters," and a flow of the dramatic narrative that is intentionally bold, symphonic, harmonious, logical, and positive.

Section 1 introduces the Journey taken by Drs. Gordon and Hall in bringing forth the first and, so far only, targeted gene delivery system, long considered the "Holy Grail of Gene Therapy". This stormy and perilous Journey taken against all odds, coveted by many, included forging through drug discovery, animal studies, first-in-human studies, orphan drug designation, fast track designation, and accelerated approval of DeltaRex-G, prevailing after a 10-year standstill with long term (12 years) cancer-free survivors, and gaining FDA authorization for "Right-to-Try" Expanded Access to DeltaRex-G for advanced pancreatic cancer, sarcoma, non-small cell lung cancer, COVID-19, cholangiocarcinoma, prostate cancer, and first-line adjuvant therapy for early stage breast cancer.

Section 2 sets the stage by traveling "off-road" into "Anaplasia" (degenerate cancer histology), conceptualized herein as the *inscrutable* "Inner Dark," that is, the outlaw territories of metastatic cancers. The DeltaRex-G nanoparticle (a tumor-targeted gene delivery vehicle) characterized as a Primal-Dinosaur Tumor-Hunter character and a

Law-Enforcer Sheriff character mounted up together as a Deputized-Dino & Sheriff Unit packing a lethal Silver Bullet (dnG1 *killer gene*).

Section 3 declares, protects, and preserves US intellectual property development in precision medicine in a strident stream-of-conscientiousness defense of continuing American innovation.

Section 4 introduces the allegory of the Hindu Durga, representing a consistent, trustworthy, and proven cancer killer (**dnG1** is a potent cyclin G1 pathway inhibitor) restoring control of the animal/cancer cell division cycle, defeating Chaos and restoring biological Law & Order by eliminating multiple bad actors (tumor cells and their accomplices) with a multi-layered approach to cancer gene therapy.

Section 5 focuses on restoring the body's natural anti-cancer immunity by repeated DeltaRex-G infusions during the course of metastatic tumor eradication.

Section 6 introduces the seminal concepts of **stem cell competence**, cell transformation, oncogene addiction, and tumor suppression in relation to biological signal transduction and the oncogenes driving subsequent gene expression. **The commanding cyclin G1/Cdk/Myc/Mdm2/p53 axis is presented as the central unifying theme of cell cycle initiation**, while linking cyclin G1 physically to p18-Hamlet (to be, or not) in the determination of cancer stem cell fate (and potential musculoskeletal regeneration).

Section 7 raises the proverbial bar for metastatic cancer survival and quality of life, documenting long-term, cancer-free survivals, thus setting a new gold standard for objective clinical responses.

Section 8 is mainly concerned with the persistent problem of "outlaw" cancer stem cells, which mediate refractoriness to conventional chemotherapies as well as the generally poor prognosis of recurrent cancers. The drama closes with a scholarly chorus of criticism regarding unproven molecular approaches to tumor targeting, outdated modes of medical thinking, and unsafe gene therapy vectors; ending with a tribute to those who worked to preserve, perfect, and restore the survival value of DeltaRex-G to the clinic.

Frederick L. Hall
Delta Next-Gene,
LLC, Santa Monica,
CA, USA

Erlinda M. Gordon
Delta Next-Gene,
LLC, Santa Monica,
CA, USA

Aveni Foundation,
Santa Monica,
CA, USA

Our Journey Beyond Sunset Boulevard: Evidence-Based Analysis of Tumor-Targeted Cancer Gene Therapy Shines a Critical Spotlight on Long-Term Cancer-Free Survival

Frederick L. Hall and Erlinda M. Gordon

Abstract

This unique "PERSPECTIVE" on *Targeted Genetic Medicine for Cancer* represents the third manuscript in a series of medical oncology papers by gene therapy pioneers, Gordon and Hall, a combined medical oncologist's and layman's trilogy recorded with the following intents and purposes: **(i) documenting significant milestones in clinical oncology for the medical community**, **(ii) honoring forthright principles of "Informed Consent"** for the advanced/*refractory* oncology patient, and **(iii) confronting logical fallacies of *popular opinion***, in light of recent critical analyses of long-term cancer-free survival data. As with the two previous historical "perspectives," the authors present noteworthy up-to-date clinical research documenting the successful management of refractory metastatic cancers with tumor-targeted gene therapy vectors—**validating "*Pathotropic*" (disease-seeking) tumor targeting *Avant la Lettre*.** This paper provides additional insights into the molecular and cellular mechanisms of both tumor-targeting and tumor-eradication. As with the prior two papers, the authors utilize the revealing powers of allegory and classic literature, adding shared iconic cinematic experiences of postmodernism at times, to educate, inform, and convey the formidable yet verifiable and important *hard-core science* (*that is, the fundamental chemistries, biophysics, molecular biology, genetics, stem cell biology, regulatory biology, synthetic virology, tumor immunology, clinical oncology, bio-pharmacology, histopathology, and cancer gene therapy*) **embodied within the "smart" therapeutic nanoparticle, DeltaRex-G: a refined "primal-hunter" & "tumor-killer"** that actively seeks out the cryptic/hidden *"Biochemical (Jailbreak) Signatures"* of metastatic cancers, delivers targeted gene therapy *"precisely"* to *tumor cells*, and ultimately *eradicates* both primary and metastatic lesions, including lymphatic metastases. Accomplishment of the *"DeltaRex-G Rescue-Mission of 2019"* with updated FDA regulatory approvals and sustainable/scalable cGMP bioproduction is considered opportune—while the **Right-to-Try** experimental therapies legislation in the United States comes face-to-face with the **U.S. FDA approval of Expanded Access for DeltaRex-G for advanced pancreatic cancer and sarcoma, and compassionate**

use for all solid tumors—as such, the authors embrace the legitimate rights of the cancer patient to be *more fully informed* of such beneficial treatments currently available in the United States.

Keywords: tumor-targeted gene therapy, cyclin G1, DeltaRex-G, cell cycle control, cancer immunotherapy

1. Introduction

> *Forty—forty—forty years ago! —ago! Forty years of continual [hunting]! forty years of privation, and peril, and storm-time! forty years on the pitiless sea! for forty years has Ahab forsaken the peaceful land, for forty years to make war on the horrors of the deep!* (**Moby Dick**, Ch.132, by Herman Melville, 1851).

Forty—forty—forty—years, added together!! Forty years of continually **hunting monsters!!** forty years of privation, and peril, and storm-time!! forty years on the pitiless sea!! for forty years have Gordon and Hall forsaken the peaceful land **to make war on the horrors of *The Deep!!*** [1, 2]. At this point, we respectfully *hoist-up* Mr. Melville's heart-rending *"Symphony,"* paraphrased, mangled, and suspended temporarily (parenthetically) in mid-air—! just as we Post-lux Postmodern Peoples must regard the "Victorian Mindset" [3] as tragically unaware and therefore largely, hugely ironic from the impeccable viewpoint of **History** which touches, embraces, and eventually reveals the *"true" nature of reality* for the world to see.

The *"true"* yet largely unaware and hugely ironic **nature of reality**—in this case —is the horrifying and yet undeniable **tragic fact:** that the Victorian sailors upon which Herman Melville crafted the Epic-Moby-Dick-Meta-Story had all admittedly expressed a collective, paralyzing fear of so-called **"cannibals:"** the savage South Pacific Islanders of the local Marquesas Islands (and the Society Islands), which misguided the shipwrecked sailors—thus the remaining lifeboats—out into open waters where *storm-time, peril, and privation* of basic human needs reached monstrous proportions—indeed, only to realize that the "cannibals" they feared most are indeed present within each and every one of us—amid "our own" natural *mob/herd* of some thirty trillion cells that make up a given **multicellular Person of Substance: You,** dear reader; **me** and **she** and **thee**.

You see, **Epictetus**, the Stoic Philosopher of ancient Greece was wise: he taught us, **"It is not Real Things that vex Humankind** (things like war, death, and/or a disease like cancer), **but Opinions of Things**.

U.S. FDA – Position Statement regarding the Federal Right-to-Try Legislation

> *"If you are interested in **Right to Try [Act/Law]**, you should discuss this pathway with your physician. Companies who develop and make drugs and biologics can provide information about whether their drug/biologic is considered an **eligible Investigational Drug** under **Right to Try** and if they are able to provide the drug/biologic under the **Right to Try Act**." – U.S. FDA 05/28/2019.*

Alas, not everyone in the medical community is celebrating your new legal **RIGHT-to-TRY an experimental therapy** [4, 5]; even an **"eligible drug,"** *one proven safe & effective in clinical trials*; even when all the conventional systemic-chemotherapy-based regimens invariably fail metastatic cancer patients: leaving prolonged side-effects, drug-resistance, and aggressive tumorsequelae in their wake

[6–8]. Thankfully, the U.S. FDA *Is-Not left dangerously out of the loop*, in regulating the translation of medical science from bench to bedside, as the pharmaceutical manufacturer's appointed bloggers [9] and the pompous parlors of Europe tend to infer as they collectively condescend [10]. Thus, celebrated **Key Opinion Leaders** differ diametrically in their *"opinions"* of your/our newly-established self-empowering legally-enforceable **Right-to-Try Legislation** (**Figure 1**).

The Most Assuring NEWS: U.S. FDA regulators with their expert reviewers of new molecular and gene-based medicines, called *"biologics,"* have long upheld a Covenant/i.e. a Code of Conduct and Protection, citing faithful compliance with exchange of information as a guiding moral imperative in our free, enlightened, self-governing postmodern society. Most assuredly, during the entire past 20-some years of the pioneering clinical development of **DeltaRex-G** (see **Figure 2**)—the first *Proactive "Tumor-Hunting/Tumor-Killing" Biomedicine* of its kind [1, 2, 15] —from tortuous depositions of the Recombinant DNA Advisory Committee (RAC) [16], to the bedsides of ≥270 advanced chemotherapy-resistant metastatic cancer patients [17–20], the FDA was ever-present and involved in the development and deployment of DeltaRex-G in the clinic:

- *providing the credibility* of U.S. **FDA R01 Funding** (*to Gordon and Hall*),

- *respectability and incentives of* **Orphan Drug Status** (*for three cancer indications*),

- *the imperatives* of **Accelerated Drug Approval for DeltaRex-G** (*former name: Rexin-G), and*

- *the expediencies* of **FDA FastTrack Designation** (*with updated cGMP compliances*)

Celebrity Opinion Leaders *vis-à-vis* Moral, Ethical, Legal Imperatives
A Cancer Patient's "Right-to-Try Act" is guided by "FDA Informed Consent"

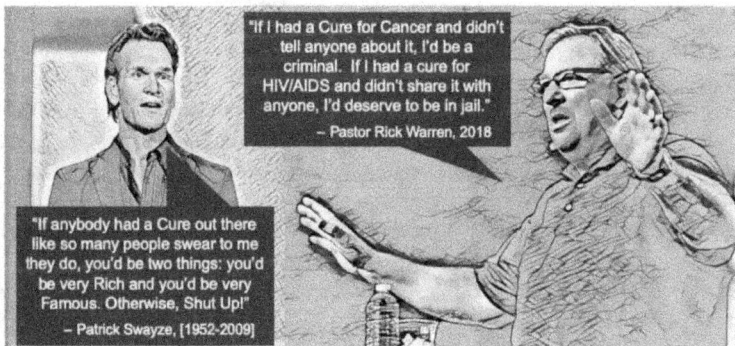

Figure 1.
Prompted & Purposeful "Opinions of Things" are often Diametrically Opposed. Good News, Folks! The jig is up; the "Third-Act" is fast upon us; the "Theatrical Clock" is metaphorically set; and the bad guys can't compete fairly in the wild-west territories of THE QUICK AND THE DEAD[f1, f2]—*which is a* Metastatic Cancer Diagnosis, *as you-all well know!! Spoiler alert: Good guys prevail with hard-core science, a duel with precision-shooting (no less), sweeping the streets clean of posers, pretenders, liars, and card-cheats with a blazing tour-de-force of bio-Logical Positivism[f3]*—**Bang!/Down**—*just like that. While bad guys collectively wrangle their own dubious reindeer games, a serious charismatic no-nonsense* "**Sheriff-Lady[f4]**" *seizes the day, faces-down the mean-spirited opposition with adamantine resolve —* **Bang!/the-Sun-shines-thru** ... *then* **Down!** — *literally,* **cinematically as it was in the movies**, *so it was on Sunset Boulevard once upon a time at the Children's Hospital of Los Angeles, 4650 Sunset Boulevard, Los Angeles, California USA[f5] [11–14].*

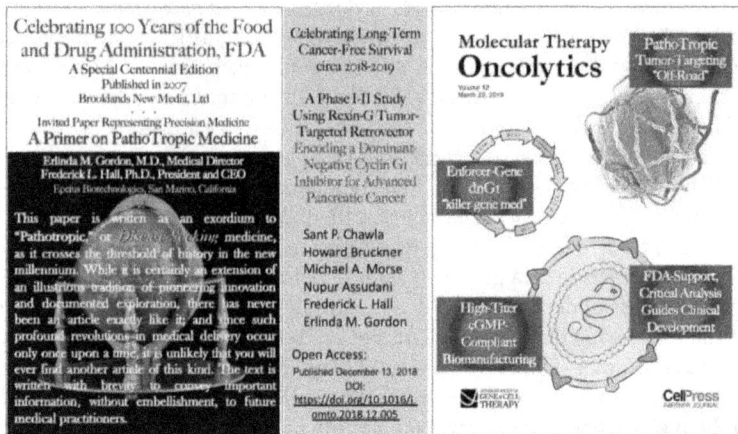

Figure 2.
Celebrating a Covenant of Trust: Revival of Tumor Targeted Gene Therapy, with U.S. FDA guidance and authorized **Sponsorship**, *as DeltaRex-G (former name: Rexin-G)—A precision gene-delivery vehicle (bearing **dnG1**, a Cyclin G1 pathway inhibitor) which actively targets the "killer gene medicine" (**dnG1** Law-ENFORCER) to metastatic lesions, beyond the vascular system, i.e., hunting Off-Road—guided deeply into metastatic tumor tissues by strong forces, molecular dynamics, and attractive high-affinities adapted from primal biochemistries to actively seek-out the cryptic histological signatures of disease. DeltaRex-G is administered i.v. repeatedly, in an attempt to meet; and safely-match (a pharmacological/mathematical* **Calculus of Parity**, *or equivalence) to eventually eliminate a given (often aggressive) chemo-resistant and increasing tumor burden.* **Clinically, DeltaRex-G provided objective benefits in hard-core chemotherapy-resistant cancers**, *and thus repeated infusions provide the late stage metastatic cancer patient with a fighting chance of achieving a clinical remission, even after chemotherapy invariably failed: thereby providing the fully-informed Stage 4* **Metastatic Cancer Patient** *with a reasonable chance of enjoying* **More Life** *and a* **Better Quality of Life** *(QOL[f6]) (see* **Figures 9** *and* **10***).*

—the U.S. FDA (and Philippine FDA, in turn) has historically honored and faithfully upheld a **Covenant of Trust** with the hapless **chemotherapy refractory Metastatic Cancer Patient**. Consequently, the *Expanded Access* to **Delta-Rex-G** and **Right-to-Try Compassionate Use** opened formally in 2019.

Indeed, (bio)actively-tumor-targeted **DeltaRex-G,** *a bona fide "Precision Medicine,"* has recently **earned ≥ 10-year Long-term-Cancer-free Survival Status**, i.e., definitive *"Curative Potential,"* based on real-world **mechanisms-of-action** and formal documentation of **long-term cancer-free survival outcomes** achieved with *Tumor-Targeted* **DeltaRex-G** —thus, a **"new gold standard"** is raised for metastatic cancer patients!

In case you missed the **NEWS Report**, it was posted on www.**CancerThera pyAdvisor**.com, on June 13, 2019, excerpted as follows [21]:

The revival of a forgotten cancer gene therapy with off the shelf potential by Cristina Bennett.

> *"A seemingly forgotten, off-the-shelf cancer gene therapy from the early 2000s appears to be getting a revival. Eight cancer patients who received the therapy a decade ago are still alive, and the features of these super responders were reported at the* ***2019 American Society of Gene and Cell Therapy*** *(ASGCT) annual meeting in Washington, D.C. And now, phase 2 trials are being planned to further evaluate the therapy."*

The tumor-targeted gene therapy, known as DeltaRex-G (formerly Rexin-G), works by delivering a retroviral vector to tumor cells that encodes for an anti-cyclin G1 construct that is meant to inhibit the cyclin G1 gene (*CCNG1*), leading to cell death. The first-in-human study was conducted in the Philippines in 2002 with patients who had chemotherapy-resistant solid tumors.

Epeius Biotechnologies Corporation, a company founded in 2004 by Frederick L. Hall, PhD, and Erlinda M. Gordon, MD, (who are also the coinventors of the therapy), sponsored the launch of several clinical trials in the United States to continue to evaluate DeltaRex-G across various chemotherapy-resistant metastatic cancer indications: **breast cancer (ClinicalTrials.gov Identifier: NCT00505271), pancreatic cancer (ClinicalTrials.gov Identifier: NCT00504998), osteosarcoma (ClinicalTrials.gov Identifier: NCT00572130), and sarcoma (ClinicalTrials.gov Identifier: NCT00505713).**

Once again, important details, as reported in a press release in August 2019:

US-FDA grants expanded access for Delta-Rex-G, A precision tumor targeted genetic medicine for metastatic cancer(s).

> *"Expanded Access for* **DeltaRex-G** *and* **Right-to-Try law** *will give individuals with different types of cancer a chance to benefit from this innovative treatment."*

Santa Monica, CA, United States, August 19, 2019/EINPresswire.com/ – **The Aveni Foundation** and the **Cancer Center of Southern California, Santa Monica CA**, are proud to announce that the **United States Food and Drug Administration has granted Expanded Access for DeltaRex-G**. This regulatory approval is based on Phase 1/2 studies demonstrating safety and efficacy for pancreatic cancer, sarcoma, and breast cancer, and long term (>10-year) survival data presented at the *American Society of Gene and Cell Therapy (ASGCT) Annual Meeting* in Washington DC.

Reporting Long-term Survival following precision tumor-targeted gene delivery to advanced chemotherapy-resistant malignancies: An Academic Milestone.

Liu et al., Molecular Therapy Vol 27(4), April 22, 2019, pg. 133. abs #275) [22].

Dr. Gordon, President of the Aveni Foundation, and Director of Biological and Immunological Therapies at the Cancer Center of Southern California, stated that "Expanded Access for DeltaRex-G and the recently-enacted **Right to Try law** will give individuals with different types of cancer a chance to benefit from this innovative treatment. DeltaRex-G is a targeted gene therapy vector that seeks the biochemical signatures (SIGs) of all invading cancers. Because the demonstrated anticancer activity of DeltaRex-G is broad spectrum, and the targeted nanoparticles display a unique (SIG)-hunting peptide, which recognizes and effectively seeks-out the tumor microenvironment, DeltaRex-G can be taken *'off the shelf,'* **clinically** – and injected intravenously over 15 minutes, without causing the side effects of chemotherapy and ungoverned immunotherapy agents."

2. Traveling *"Off-Road"* into *"Anaplasia"*: the metastatic *"Inner Dark"* DeltaRex-G: a primal cancer-hunter & tumor-killer, from a conceptual point of view

Here, we will need to *grasp* the concept of a **"Primal Hunter:"** age-old (evolutionarily speaking) **"Designer-Dinosaurs"** (as artfully drawn by Mr. Shaun Keenan), with their natural (primal) dog-like/horse-like sensibilities *"to-Track Bad-Actors Off-Road,"* beyond the vascular highways, and even *"further Off-Road"* into an uncharacterized *wilderness* (**Figure 3**): tracking, hunting, mapping the *"Inner Dark"* (undefined properties) of diseased tissues, where even timid (anergic, i.e., repressed/intimidated) white blood cells fear-to-tread (*you'll see*). Only then, can one separate conceptually the **Primal-Dino-Hunter**

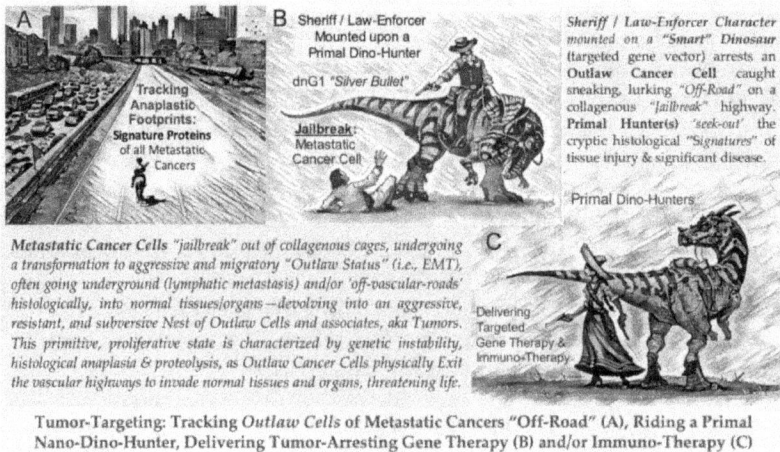

Tumor-Targeting: Tracking *Outlaw Cells* of Metastatic Cancers "Off-Road" (A), Riding a Primal Nano-Dino-Hunter, Delivering Tumor-Arresting Gene Therapy (B) and/or Immuno-Therapy (C)

Figure 3.
Allegory of Sheriff/Law-Enforcer with Killer-Gene-Medicine Riding a Nano-Dino. Rendered with iconic drama, pathos, and suspense of a postmodern Western Movie (A), complete with real-world **hunting/ tracking** *of telltale 'Signatures of Metastatic-Disease'*— in reality, **cryptic and hidden** *yet biochemically discernable anaplastic (devolved) signatures of "exposed" collagenous proteins, revealing secondary and tertiary structural conformations, which are biochemically-sensed, i.e., attracted by forces acting at a distance, i.e.,* "Hunted," *(though non-covalently-bound) by the phylogenetically ancient yet highly-conserved D2 propeptide domain of von Willebrand Factor, as described by Gordon and Hall [23–26]. In this theatrical/allegorical manner, the concept of the* **Deputized-Dino-Hunter** *(the targeted gene vector) is separable from the* **Therapeutic Payload** *(the cancer gene therapy)—in this case, the* **Sheriff/Law-Enforcer Character (B)** *bears a* **Killer Gene Medicine** *(dominant-negative dnG1 construct), while the two-fisted gunslinger lady,* **Sheriff/Law-Enforcer Character (C)** *delivers a strategic combination of targeted* dnG1 *Gene-Therapy and* targeted *Immuno-Therapy which seeks to arrest and/or destroy* **"Outlaw" Cancer Cells** *and their cellular accomplices.*

(the *tumor-targeted gene delivery vehicle*) from the **Sheriff (Law-Enforcer)** charac-ters, **with their** therapeutic *Silver Bullets* (genetic *"payloads"* of tumor-busting fire-power). Mounted-up together—**as a Dino & Sheriff Unit, packing the lethal "dnG1 *killer gene*"** construct—DeltaRex-G is a *synthetic* tumor-targeted **cancer-gene-therapy vector**, i.e., a *medicinal nanoparticle* administered intravenously (*i.v.*) to seek-out and eradicate advanced metastatic cancers.

In this picturesque first chapter, we recount the first voyages of Gordon and Hall into the cavernous/cancerous *Inner Dark* of diseased tissues, wherein the caution-ary words **"Hic Sunt Dracones"** *(Here be Dragons)* that once echoed in the History of Exploration, resound within the solemn missions and accomplishments of the U.S. Food and Drug Administration. The main point being, that there are *indeed* ways for modern science and medicine to proceed in dark, scary (unknown) territories— **that is, with due caution and resolve, with faithful recording of methods, results, clinical insights, interim analyses, and with rigorous analytics regard-ing patient outcomes** [1, 2]. For our intentionally-theatrical and instructional pur-poses, we will simply *"Deputize"* these **Primal-Dino-Hunters**—found metaphorically *sniffing/hunting/mapping-out* **Outlaw-trails** *amidst the collagenous corpses, skeletons, gristle, and biochemistries of our primal Pre-Cambrian past.* As shown in **Figure 3B** and **C**, the **Deputized Dino-Hunters** (tumor-targeted vectors) will even NOW enable oncologists to "Hunt-down" the corrupted/transformed mean-spirited (DNA-damaged) **"Outlaw Cancer Cells"** that are caught in the fla-grant *Lawless Act of behaving Badly*: that is, aggressive *Outlaw* Cancer Cells, *along with their Protective Supportive Enabling* **Cellular Entourages and Accom-plices,** are seen traveling and wildly-proliferating *"Off-Road"* in a histologically-distressed state of chaos & disarray—that is, a benighted **state of *Anaplasia*** (degenerate histopathology), which is a particularly badass characteristic of advanced metastatic cancers and disease progression.

Cancer Metastasis—defined as the spread of malignant cells to distant sites —is the primary cause of death when standard treatments fail to produce durable clinical responses. The theory of "**Tumor Dormancy**" was originated to account for clinical findings of cancer recurrence (relapse) long after surgical removal of the primary tumors [27, 28]; thereby characterizing "metastatic tumor dormancy" — including (i) immunological dormancy, (ii) angiogenic dormancy [29], and/or (iii) cancer cell dormancy [7, 30]— as physiological mechanisms of drug resistance which continue to thwart conventional cytotoxic cancer therapies. During the past 20 years, the *supportive* and *protective role* of the *tumor microenvironment* in cancer progression has grown beyond Outlaw-cancer-cells *taking blood vessels* (vascular endothelial cells) *hostage*, to include both **Tumor-Associated Immune Cells** (e.g., **TAMs**; [31]) and **Cancer-Associated Fibroblasts (CAFs**; [32]) as unwitting accomplices "hijacked" in the outlaw/metastatic process. That is: CAFs and TAMs are currently viewed as *abettors of tumor progression at the crossroads of (malignant) Epithelial-to-Mesenchymal Transition (EMT) and chemotherapy resistance* [6]; thereby providing mechanistic links between tumor recurrence, daunting drug resistance, **CAF** dynamics, **TAM** interactions, and the dynamic nature of the **Collagenous Extracellular Matrix** (Col-ECM) scaffolds found within the *Reactive Stroma* of metastatic lesions [33]. The changing mechanistic view(s) of cancer recurrence, cancer biology, tumor drivers, treatment strategies, and chemo-refractoriness are highlighted by the following 'cutting-edge' commentary:

"It is commonly accepted that disseminated tumour cells (DCTs) survive cytotoxic chemotherapy because they are not proliferating. A new study now finds that, in contrast to this long-standing concept, **both the dormant and proliferative cancer cells are protected from chemotherapy when they reside at the perivascular niche**" [34].

Indeed, the identification of such cancer-associated chemotherapeutically-challenged "**niche**"compartments may indeed engender many new ECM-directed strategies, perchance to *"eradicate DTCs and prevent metastasis"* in some far-distant future of medicine [8]; however, the tumor-targeting, i.e., "**Pathotropic**" (literally *disease seeking*) "**lesion-defining studies**" of Gordon & Hall circa 2000–2020, are instructive: by purposefully inventing/refining/defining **proactive "lesion-seeking"nanoparticles** incorporating a physiological *Tumor-Surveillance Function*—derived by molecular engineering the primal D2 propeptide domain (i.e., "tail-end") of von Willebrand Factor (vWF-D2; [23–26]—they embarked upon a pioneering approach to "**Map**" the *"Tierra Incognita"*of cancer's *metastatic Inner Dark* [1, 2]; thereby sailing forth intently, purposefully, to deliver the goods to refractory patients in the cancer clinics, as you will see for yourself ... *by the end of this timely paper.*

If you followed this reasoning, you will realize that **the *Outlaw* Cancer Cells aren't really *Sleeping* at all** (unless, of course, they advantageously decide to do so) —**they are *Hiding! Lurking!*** Just like the *"Bad Actors"* of the proverbial **Wild West**, cancer cells have traveled back in evolutionary time (to single-cellularity); they have passed nearly-naked through the proverbial (vascular) *"hole in the wall,"* traveling *way **Off-Road*** beyond the reach of current medical (immunological) therapies into the perilous **Outlaw-infested** and ill-defined **state of *Anaplasia* (Figure 4)**. What are we waiting for? Grab a Picturesque **Nano-Dino-Hunter** of your very own, and let's track down some metastatic **Bad Actors**, *together*—for now you have FDA-permissions, tumor-targeting maps, and Right-to-Try Legislation in your favor for the first time in history: But let's be cautious, principled, alert!!! Remember, this is *Tombstone Territory*.

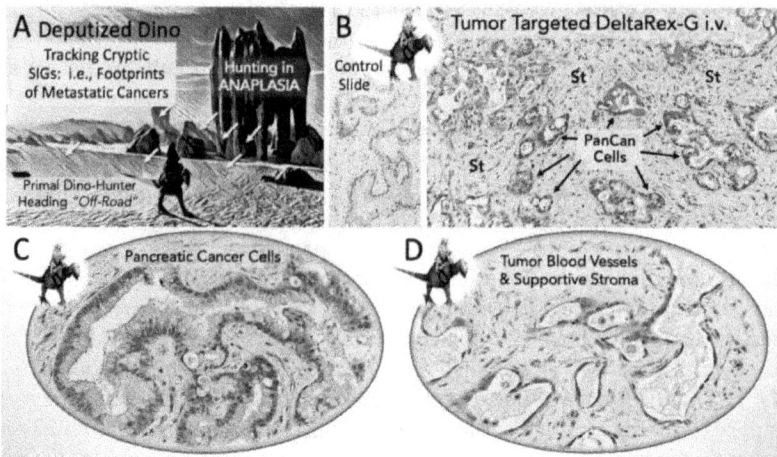

Figure 4.
Allegory of the Deputized-Dino translated to the level of Histology and Cancer Cell Biology. (A):
Deputized Nano-Dino with a mounted Sheriff (dnG1 gun-wielding) Law-Enforcer shown here heading
"Off-road," tracking cryptic SIGs (discernible biochemical footprints) in the perilous pathological state of
"Anaplasia." Turning microscopically to actual human pancreatic cancer tissues obtained by surgical biopsy
following intravenous infusions of tumor-targeted DeltaRex-G as cancer gene therapy (B-D): Specific
histochemical staining for the targeting moiety (envelope protein) of the "smart" nanoparticle, viewed under a
microscope, versus control slides (inset, in B), reveals "Three Cellular Targets" identified within the flagrant
metastatic tumor: (i) robust Pancreatic Cancer Cells (B, enlarged in C), and their characteristic hostages,
including (ii) proliferative Tumor Vasculature (brown stain of elongate endothelial cells, enlarged in D)
and accomplices (iii) Cancer-Associated Fibroblasts (TAFs, TAMs, brown stain) imbedded in dense fibrous
(desmoplastic) connective tissues including cellular elements and extracellular matrix (ECM) and collagenous
proteins referred to as the Stroma (St) of a solid tumor.

3. Badges of responsibility, innovation, and intellectual properties

Notice to all Interested Americans: *"Badges? Ya'll Ain't Got No (IP-)Badges?!"*
First Point to Consider: not everyone has FDA permissions to hunt-down *Bad Actors* in the **Wild West**, nor to inject 100 billion *smart* tumor-targeted nanoparticles into the vein a human cancer patient [1, 2]. In addition to a U.S. FDA-sanctioned, i.e., **Deputized-Dino**, with its requisite sponsorship, regulatory over-sight(s), cGMP protocols, and rules of engagement in place; anyone seeking *The Treasures of the Sierra Madre* knows that you will need to have solid **Intellectual Property "Badges"** (IP-Badges) in this fierce biotechnology space. **Shiny-new IP-Badges**—known as 'wealth-gathering instruments' to biotech bounty hunters—hold a hefty weight of status, tradition, and responsibility which often places the individual hunters/healers at odds with the biopharmaceutical collective as a whole. Circa September 2018, Hall and Gordon received *sad NEWS*: After trailblazing solid-state wound/bone healing from molecule to medicine [35–38], capturing/revealing primitive stem cells for regenerative medicine and gene therapy applica-tions [39–41], targeting pharmaceutical agents to injured tissues [42], and develop-ing the world's first precision targeted gene delivery platform to be validated in the cancer clinic [15–22]—that is to say, *after* Gordon and Hall had coauthored (i.e., taught) > 150 issued patents—they were informed by US Patent examiners (of final action) that being: *"enough is enough,"* after 150 some definitive proofs-of-principle describing and developing evidence-based inventions, all successfully reduced to practice, they were informed that the *entire oeuvre* of their enabling/disruptive/clinically-effective *Pathotropic Platform Biotechnologies* would simply be *Assimilated* —thus, **no new IP-Badges for Ya'll!**

> *"We are the Borg. Lower your shields and surrender your ships. We will add your biological and technological distinctiveness to our own. Your culture will adapt to service us. Resistance is futile."*
>
> — The Borg, *(Star Trek: First Contact).*

Fortunately, Hall et al. realized the importance of **continued U.S. innovation in Pathotropic (disease-seeking) tumor-targeting** as a Cornerstone of Precision Drug Delivery for Oncology, not to mention pro-active tumor surveillance and targeted theragnostic (*therapeutics* with *diagnostic*) applications. At this pivotal point in our journey, when it's all about *saving people, hunting things*, we'll simply *listen-in* to the *IP-Lawyer-Scrimmage* — as Dr. Hall outlines a so-called *"Hail-Mary pass"* in the sandlot, for lack of a more descriptive metaphor (see **Figure 5**). **No worries, *this time we win*:** Hall et al. prevailed; a new U.S. "Pathotropic" (tumor-targeting) Patent issued in the springtime of 2019: i.e., **"We *won* your official IP-Badges! For ya!"**

Dr. Hall's explanatory letter to *Fish & Richardson P.C.* (representing Hall & Gordon), in addition/concert with academic interests at USC) regarding *tacit patent office rejection* of the latest intellectual property claim/request for new updated/authorized **IP-Badges**!

"Dear Todd et al.:

Here is our "spiral-bound" *Pass* that will lead you into the medical, biotechno-logical, and legal End-Zone (of American Medical History) for a solid six points in the final waning moments ...

Counterpoint Biomedica LLC (a partnership with purpose) represents a turning point in Medical History (*get ready*)—we at Counterpoint Biomedica LLC already know that—and yet you don't know that YET—and that's OK/good for us (no one does).

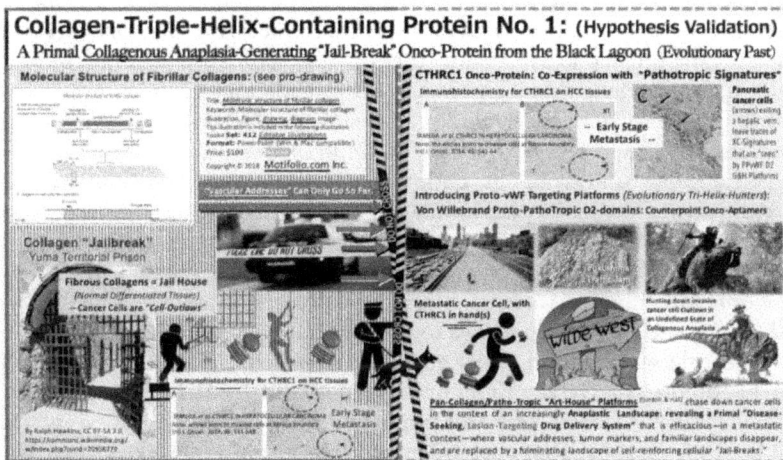

Figure 5.
Hypothesis Validation: Concordance with destructive Outlaw Cancer Cell EMT/Behavior. The Storyboard—*Self-serving aka Outlaw-cells "breaking-out" of fibrous (collagenous) conformity; once* off-road, *the Outlaw cancer cells begin expressing then dropping CTHRC1, a collagen-triple-helix-repeat-containing-protein: i.e., a "Jail-break" (Anaplasia-generating)* **onco-protein**, *which "incites" proteolytic* **ECM-deformations**, *hence biochemical conformational (secondary and tertiary distortions),* **Signatures of Anaplasia** *(vWF-D2-recognized SIGs). Apparently, the above "storyboard figure," together with Dr. Hall's letter, served to convince (technically, "teach") the conscientious U.S. patent examiners: New* **IP Badges** *were formally "issued" in mid-2019.* **Grasped thematically, or in intricate, gristly biochemical details,** *the CTHRC1 "JailBreak" oncoprotein is timely, medically important, and logically related to the* **Outlaw Cell behavior** *and* **escape** *into the (empirically uncharted)* **state of Anaplasia**. *Thus, Hall & Gordon prevailed with definitive innovation, experimentation, quantification, validation, & clinical documentation.*

At this point, we would like (and are duly encouraged) to take a thoughtfully considered position: STASIS IN THE MEDICAL ARTS IS TANTAMOUNT TO DEATH!! Thus, we are encouraged to Defend the Intellectual Property Rights of the Originating Inventors (Hall and Gordon) who thought and drove the seminal and productive **Concepts of Patho-Tropic Disease Hunting** (*i.e., disease-seeking medicine that is functionally, physiologically, medically; and not IYI/academically Collagen-Binding Armchair-defined*) forward Intellectually—in the crucible of human disease—to single-handedly pioneer an entirely new field of medicine (*i.e., the Actual/not-merely Hypothetical/Theoretical*), and by so doing, we have revealed the ***Primal Face of Pathology*** (Primitive Collagenous Anaplasia) and have pioneered the *entire field* of **PathoTropic Medicine**, *Avant La Lettre*.

As such, "*In Saving People, Hunting with Primitive Things,*" we have fulfilled the postmodern promise of **Precision Medicine**, as well as the goal of the **USC Norris Cancer Cente**r (*to make cancer a disease of the past*), as well as the motto of ***Supernatural,*** the postmodern TV series. Seriously Todd, in light of the reviewers (hollow *and yet chilling*) claims of "obviousness,"—of our Brand NEW Artful stone tools, as we evolved/engineered a once-useless fragment of biochemical pre-history yet again into a Useful Enabling Platform after Useful Enabling Platform (**Note: not one, but > 150 IPs**)—curiously, it's like we *The True Pioneers* are now suddenly playing an "away-game"—even with F&R—and I/we wonder why this is (?); thus, we must now take a more strident, principled, and scholarly stand, as you will see.

Frankly: they (experts) cannot have/steal what they don't yet understand; and they can't/don't yet understand it, until they acknowledge the utility/**design-engineering superiority** of a given **Drug-Delivery Platform** (accordingly, with *transient* IP rights; i.e. a better mousetrap, a new utility patent). **In Performing our own Interim Analysis** of what these 'so-called obvious' Onco-Aptamers (synthetic peptides) we designed with an ability to seek and find the fabric of nature and thus human disease .... (*note: without the regulatory complexities active proteins, viruses, genes or vaccines being involved*), we realize that the **Onco-Aptamer platform**—in addition to targeting monoclonal antibodies (mAbs) and/or Taxol or microRNAs, or anything and everything that is an obvious drug at any time in the future—yet we know now, by our own medical, clinical, **Physiological analysis**, that the "Onco-aptamer Probes" Themselves (*you know, the Superior Ones that are brighter in the mouse*) are a Proof-of-Principle for both future "**Diagnostics**" and "**Tumor Spotting**"/removing CTCs/preventing DTCs/and Lymphatic Diagnostics—**which we hereby Claim for the American People, who supported us all along.**

Thus, **the Exhibit** (attached White Paper) is a composite **History of Pathotropic Medicine** (as we lived it); as you will see; it is intended to be a ***Formal Moral, Legal, and Ethical Challenge*** to the predatory patent trolls intent on commandeering/warehousing future gene-based medicine ... with our **Triumphant Vision of Hypothesis-Driven Evidence-Based Medically-Relevant Physiologically-Validated New and Important "Art-House Engineering" Optimized for New Medical/Diagnostic Applications** ... for things like simple, or not so simple, **Precision Diagnostics.** The intention (legal strategy) is to go all out, spare no expense—come what may—for the future of medicine, indeed the precision medicines we made, and the precision diagnostics, and all the precision biomedical engineering of your children and your children's children, might just depend upon what we few stand for today.

Basically, it is very important to realize here on in, that it was not the static **Collagen Binding-Bandages** Hall et al. invented long ago, *but the Saving-People Hunting-Things IDEA*, i.e., the possible clinical potential (***Hypothesis***) of a primal pan-tropic collagen "**Hunter**" **from the black lagoon** that just might travel further than the blood vessels into the degenerate and shifting landscape of cancerous disease—Interim analysis, working hypothesis, thus evidence-based medicine; a far cry from [theoretical] "armchair speculation". The White Paper is an attempt to share candidly [with professionals, lawyers, oncologists, committees only].

You see, Todd, what we (Hall & Gordon) did, was much more than make static bandages/medicines—we thought about possibilities of deeper penetration into tumors than blood vessels via exposed-ECM-deep targeting; we realized Pan-tropic would be *medically superior (even I couldn't guess which collagen types, where?)*, and went to work on the "useless" cast-away, admittedly lower-affinities of the vWF-D2 domain ... by creative engineering, bio-engineering; necessarily, creatively, SHAPING each *biologically perverse* (new utility, platform, viral envelope, peptide, etc.) clinical application, each new D2-shaped-platform; each, a new engineering challenge... yet with the solid scientific assurance that what we did with the Counterpoint Onco-Aptamer Platform (better than previous Bv1 = invention), was to provide **a Bright New Tool for Diagnosis**, reaching and thereby reporting cancers in the lymphatics (diagnosis), as well as treating and even curing human disease with many patented vector designs etc. In the fullness of time, this PrimalPanCollagen-Hunter (Hall&Gordon-D2Arthouse probes), which shed its Bright Proto-Promethean Light upon the Nature of Disease—for the first time in history—revealing the distorted and largely undefined collagenous landscapes of our diseased tissues which have been eroded and deformed by significant disease (Note: added and abetted by a Primal Collagenous (triple helical) "collagenous Jail-Break" Oncoprotein (CTHRC1: recently discovered, *to this prescient Inventor's delight*. See Zhang et al., 2014, Molecular Carcinogenesis 54:1554–1566) which is linked to promotion of cancer metastasis at-large by the dynamic distortions (proteolysis of collagens) that generate/espouse the primitive degenerative, anaplastic territories and outlaw trails of metastatic cancer cells). Alas, it is also important to note that such bold **Promethean endeavors** (bold challenge to arrogant authority), often require **Herculean resolve**: that being well-prepared, well-intended IP lawyers with a good pair of hands in the end zone ... with due caution to all involved that **the *judgement of history is impeccable.***

Cheers, and go deep, we got this one! PS: Spiral-bound refers to concordant publication of White Paper Content/Bio-logic in a prominent peer-reviewed Journal.

Rick.

Attachment: Slide Deck [DeltaRex-G White Paper] Exhibit – available as historical medical archives.

Enter, The Jailbreak Onco-Protein: *Collagen-Triple-Helix-Repeat-Containing Protein #1* (**CTHRC1**), recently discovered, important conceptually; and **like CCNG1/(Cyclin G1** gene) [20], initially found to be highly (transiently) expressed in models of **vascular restenosis** *(cellular hyperplasia),* in intimate association with the migratory behavior and the proliferative cell cycle control programs of myofibroblastic (neo-intimal) cells of injured blood vessels [43]. Soon after its molecular-genetic discovery, the *CTHRC1* gene product was identified as a biologically dangerous secreted, *oncogenic protein*, aka an "**Oncoprotein**" operating in the **Anaplastic** *tombstone territories* [44]: specifically, CTHRC1 expression appears to be directly—both *aberrantly up-regulated and mechanistically linked*—to the initial breakout, clearly a *Collagen-Jailbreak*, both enabling and resulting-in **Cancer Metastasis (in Allegory, the *Jailbreak* and *Escape* of Outlaw cancer cells),** driving the Outlaw-formation of human solid tumors: including metastatic melanoma, hepatocellular carcinoma, and advanced metastatic cancers of the colon, stomach, breast, ovaries, lungs, thyroid gland, and pancreas [45–47]. By driving/up-regulating the major *"Architectural"* ECM-remodeling enzyme activities—the elite cadres of "ECM-digesting and deforming Matrix-*Metallo*-"*Proteases*" [48], which tailor, shape, remodel, thus *transform Collagenous Landscapes* histologically by signaling/prompting/sculpting collagenous matrix proteins, expressly for self-centered *tumorigenic* purposes [49, 50]. **Outlaw Cancer Cells** utilize the "Jail-break"-CTHRC1-Oncoprotein ruthlessly: (i) to recruit and commandeer TAFs into the degenerative process [51], **(ii)** to stifle TAMs and suppress the cancer patient's local immune responses [49], and **(iii)** to whip-up normal budding vascular endothelial cells into a neovascular frenzy [52]; thereby creating a pernicious DNA-damaged band of self-motivated, self-renewing **Cancer Cells** undergoing progressive Epithelial to Mesenchymal Transition (EMT) to *Off-Road motility and mobility*; which, together with their band of *intimidated* cellular accomplices (taken-hostage), drive unbridled metastatic tumor formation [53]—viewed allegorically, and yet observed objectively, histologically as a cadre of armed and dangerous *Outlaw Cancer Cells and Accomplices operating dangerously, flagrantly, aggressively in a degenerate state of Anaplasia* (see **Figures 4–6**).

Ordinarily, anatomic arrays of "fibrillar" collagen proteins form the structural basis/scaffolds of organs and tissues, including vasculature, bone, sinews, and tendons such that there exists a vast constellation of "cryptic" sequences, orderly helical configurations, and/or discernable collagenous conformations *hidden* within the primary, secondary, and/or tertiary structures of the organized collagen-fibril-rich matrices, which require structural trauma and/or significant disease, and/or site-specific proteolysis for cryptic collagenous signatures to become histologically/*Pathologically "Exposed"* [54–56]. Indeed, high-resolution electron microscopy and optical imaging is able to characterize the *appearance* of **tumor-associated collagen signatures** (TACs) associated with the tumor-stroma interface at the metastatic invasion front [57]; remarkably, high-throughput proteomic screening was able to

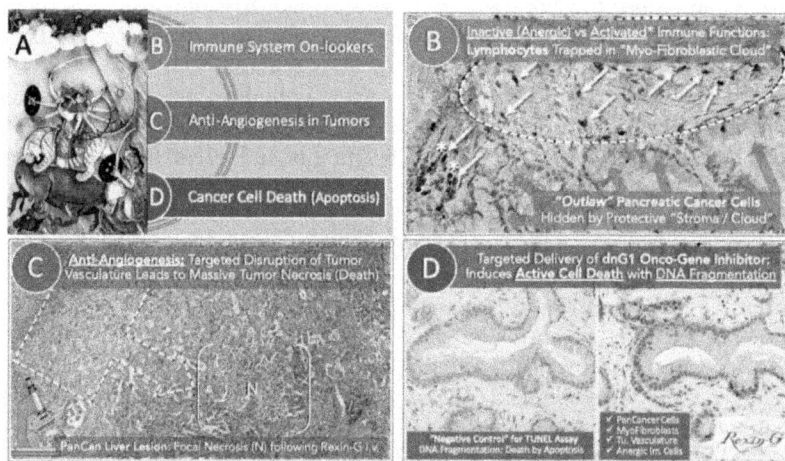

Figure 6.
The Multi-talented Goddess Durga fighting [and slaying] Mahishasura, the buffalo-demon: Hindu
Mythology, *(A)*, is an appropriate Allegory for *DeltaRex-G operating mechanistically on* **Multiple
Histological Levels** *within flagrant metastatic tumors of a pancreatic cancer patient, as seen here in a surgical
tumor biopsy after* **DeltaRex-G** *i.v. (B-D).* **Breaking/Arresting Immunological Indifference** *(aka*
Immune Anergy, *B) including "creepy" Tumor-Associated myoFibroblastic (TAF) accomplices, which form
a protective "Cloud" (Desmoplastic Stroma) surrounding the Cancer cells;* **Anti-Angiogenesis is evident:**
*Breaking/Arresting Tumor Neo-Vascularization (C) by slashing tumor-enslaved/proliferative vascular
endothelial cells, resulting in massive downstream destruction of tumor tissues in a* Showdown *known in
histological circles as "focal necrosis" (N, brackets). Biochemically, the tumor-targeted delivery of the "Enforcer
Gene" (dnG1) blocks the Cyclin G1-mediated cell activation/survival pathway, resulting in "cell death" with
telltale DNA-fragmentation—Apoptosis: Boom/Down! Tumor Cell Death!* The brownish TUNEL staining
for **DNA fragments** confirms massive apoptosis, eradication of cellular 'Bad Actors,'—the tumor appears like
'Boot Hill,' shown here histologically (D) in pancreatic cancer cells, accomplice myo-fibroblastic (i.e., stromal
elements), tumor neo-vasculature, and anergic immune cells, thus reducing the tumor mass.*

identify a quasi-myriad of so-called *cryptic protein binding sites* and have provided a veritable potpourri: specifically, a *"Proteomic Protein Data Set"* of some 152 candidate protein targets associated with malignant desmoplasias at the *cancer invasion front*, including daunting type-specific collagen-type protein expressions and about 22 unique so-called "myo-fibroblastic signatures" [58]. In contrast to bio-panning and random screening for putative clues amid such a disheartening array of prospective dynamic molecular complexities, Hall & Gordon thoughtfully considered and engaged the physiological hence clinical utility of a **"Smart"** (i.e., **tumor-targeted) vWF-D2-derived nanoparticle, A 'Primal Pan-tropic Tri-Helix-Hunter'** [23–26]—FDA-deputized and unleashed to **Map-Out the Outlaw-Territories**. The **FDA-deputized Nano-Dino-Hunter** from our evolutionary past is *an adaptively-engineered, artfully-designed, minimalistic, biocompatible,* vWF^{D2}-derived, *experimentally optimized and selected* "HUNTER" *aka* **gene therapy vector** deployed clinically: **(i)** to map-out out the biochemical **Tierra Incognita of OUR histological** *Inner Dark;* **(ii)** to deliver precision **Cancer Gene Therapy** (with increased safety, efficacy, outcomes) to human metastatic cancers [59]. At the time, it was a road less traveled:

"In the course of scientific research and development it is often "The Road Not Taken," that is, the conscious decision to take the road less traveled by, that turns out to make the most significant difference in terms of historical outcome. In the case of targeted gene delivery, it was the conscious decision to target a common histopathological property of the metastatic process, rather than the unique and ever-changing surface features (ligands, receptors, etc.) of the individual cancer cells, that made all the difference in terms of enhancing the efficiency of tumor-targeting under the most demanding of physiological conditions. Indeed, in the process of metastasis and metastatic tumor formation, both nascent and underlying extracellular matrix (ECM) proteins are characteristically exposed; and it is this characteristic exposure of one particular class of ECM proteins, the ubiquitous and determinative collagens (i.e., collagen patefacio, from Gordon & Hall, 2009), that now forms the basis for disease-seeking (or Pathotropic) tumor targeting" [19]).

4. Targeting the multi-dimensional ECM with DeltaRex-G *i.v*

Cancer Cells & Accomplices *"Bite the Dust"* **The Enforcer: dnG1** – *Bang/Down: Apoptosis!*

Survival, Evasion, Resistance, and Escape (SERE) —Militant aspects of metastatic cells, tumor formation, and disease progression which continue to confound conventional cancer therapies:

- The stifling, intimidation, and coercion of stromal fibroblasts and immune cells; turning innocent bystanders into accomplices in the *metastatic jailbreaks* [6, 60–65].

- The chemical coercion and vascular endothelial cells (with secreted growth factors) into a frenzy of vascular cell proliferation (neo-angiogenesis), producing abundant tumor neo-vasculature, which provides the rationale for *anti-angiogenic tumor therapies* [66, 67].

- The shifting genetic identity (genotype) and epithelial-mesenchymal plasticity (EMT) of cancer cells [68, 69]—with empirical cancer mutation rates from ~50 mutations/tumor (breast, pancreatic cancer) to upwards of 100–200 mutations/tumor (melanoma and lung cancer—is a very serious problem biologically and strategically: *"Consequently, making decisions on such evolving high rates of mutations in human solid tumors make these approaches fraudulent ('molecular false flags') and irresponsible as evident from the high failure outcomes of (so called) molecular target"* [68].

Consequently, we will need to invoke another **Dramatic Allegory** to proceed safely: in this case, the protective/restorative blessings of the fierce, powerful, notably invincible aspects of the revered **Goddess Durga** of the Hindu pantheon, whose mythological/intellectual function is to fight and to creatively overcome such unruly demons: as depicted in **Figure 6A**). In this case, the blue-colored buffalo demon represents the allegorical/histological *Outlaw* $^{DNA-Damaged}$ **cancer cell**, amid a myo-fibroblastic *cloud* (desmoplastic stroma) of **cytological hostages**, *immune-system on-lookers,* and vascularizing accomplices (tumor angiogenesis), which threaten the stability of the 'cosmos.' The invincible, ever-resourceful **Mounted Durga shows a** *Decisive Multi-Pronged Approach:* (**i**) to restore *anergic* (timid) immune responses, (**ii**) to destroy supportive *tumor-associated vasculature,* and (**iii**) to directly *eliminate the rogue cancer cells (i.e., the blue buffalo demon)* which are selfishly, flagrantly driving cancer metastasis. Characteristically, **the Durga** is inaccessible; yet she is always triumphant in extreme situations, *with just the right tool for the job,* as she brings with her a dominating weapon: Dominant-Negative Cyclin G1 Blocker (**dnG1**): an expression construct (*Silver Bullet*) embodied within the tumor-targeted **DeltaRex-G nanoparticle**—a proven cancer killer, as **Cyclin G1** function is a powerful *"Survival Factor"* and a *pivotal driver* of many if not most **advanced cancers** [20]. Thus, the **Allegorical Durga** depicted in **Figure 6** is packing a consistent, trustworthy, and proven cancer killer: [**dnG1** is a potent **Cyclin G1 Pathway Inhibitor**] restoring *control of the cell division cycle*; defeating chaos and *restoring bodily Law & Order* by eliminating multiple *Bad Actors* (cancer cells, accomplices) with a *Multi-layered approach* to cancer gene therapy.

5. Therapeutically restoring the body's innate anti-cancer immunity

Breaking Immune Anergy (*Indifference*)—The Gristly Gist of Drug Resistance.

Targeting the Tumor Microenvironment (TME) in an attempt to improve chemotherapeutic efficacy, perchance to modulate drug resistance, is a *"modern trend"* in medical oncology [69–72]. Renewed interest in the TME notwithstanding, numerous attempts at combining *ungoverned* chemotherapy with *unguided* immunotherapy have been hampered, often stymied, by off-target side-effects which consistently lead to rather serious clinical adverse events:

"A significant fraction of patients treated with chemo-immunotherapy exhibited immune-related adverse events of grade 3 (moderate-to-severe symptoms) or higher (life-threatening-symptoms), with a 10-20% rate of treatment discontinuation owing to severe adverse events associated with chemoimmunotherapy" [72–75]. **This highlights the problem of off-target toxicity and the need to develop targeted and localized delivery systems** [72].

The **Anaplastic TME**, with its *mercurial* and *diverse* collagenous exo-architectures, dynamic extracellular "matrix" (ECM) proteins, and its *wildly complicated, rapidly-evolving* (genetically-shifty) cadre of badass **"outlaw" cancer cells**, intimidated immune cell hostages & accomplices, reactive secretory fibroblasts, supportive vascular endothelial cells, and associated microvascular pericytes is a rude, impertinent, and largely **"Unmapped Territory"** at the sub-cellular level: that is, at the hard-core physicochemical nature of reality—save for the *"first, and so far only"* [15] disease-seeking clinical *devices and investigations* of

Gordon & Hall—brandishing **DeltaRex-G,** a broad-spectrum *Pathotropic*$^{vWF-D2}$ nanoparticle **bearing dnG1,** a *"Killer Gene"* delivered intravenously *(i.v.)* in clinical trials with advanced metastatic cancers [1, 2].

Upon intravenous injection, 300 billion *smart* tumor-targeted nanoparticles rapidly traverse the human heart, and the lungs, and the heart once again as an *"Armed-Posse"* of mounted **Nano-Dino-Hunters** (bearing *dnG1-Inhibitor* gene therapy) charge off into the rapids of the systemic circulation—*guided by Primal Pan-tropic working relationships* [i.e., **vWF-D2: lesion-seeking affinities** [23–26] —aiming to *seek-out-and-arrest* and/or *shoot-to-destroy* the entire proliferative population of *cancerous Bad Actors* in each and every one of your **primary, occult, nascent, or advanced, growing, dormant, and/or genetically- and phenotypically- progressing metastatic cancer lesions** —thereby restoring normal histology with precision gene delivery *(specifically, tumor-targeted* **dnG1 gene delivery***)*, restoring **Cellular** *Law-and-Order* (Genetic/DNA fidelity—*'twas lost along with natural p53- mediated tumor suppression*), which favors & endorses "**You,**" dear reader: namely, your personal harmonious multicellularity.

Importantly, by targeting and eliminating the entire supporting cast of *cancerous Bad Actors lurking* within the **Tumor Microenvironment** (TME), Gordon & Hall observed and reported (upon painstaking interim analyses) "**A Return of Innate Anti-Cancer Immunity,**" *a cellular saving grace,* if you would; as overt immune activity is clearly participating **biologically, i.e., histologically** (*in the absence of chemotherapy-related immune-suppression*) **in the process of tumor eradication and the establishment of clinical remissions**. Critical analysis of preclinical studies in experimental animals [19, 73–75], followed by a progression of clinical trials in humans [17–22, 76–78], served both to validate and to optimize the clinical utility of **"Pathotropic Targeting"** for the management of advanced metastatic cancers. The demonstrated *Physiological Cancer Surveillance Function* embodied in the **DeltaRex-G nanoparticle** is exceedingly efficient, selective, genetically precise, and clinically advantageous. Empirically, the *bioactive selectivity* (high-affinities) *for cancerous tissues and the quantitative pharmacokinetics* are (**i**) **sufficiently rapid** (minutes), (**ii**) **sufficiently efficient** in terms of tumor penetrance (extensive), (**iii**) **sufficiently selective** for proliferative target cells (many), and (**iv**) **sufficiently potent** in terms of demonstrating dose-dependent single-agent anti-cancer bioactivity to perform so well as a monotherapy! Consequently, the observed physiological tumor-targeting cancer surveillance function is compelling enough to consider, envisage, achieve, and document the long-standing goal and objective of *tumor eradication* (aka **objective clinical efficacy**), even in advanced chemotherapy-resistant metastatic cases, with concomitant improvements in **QoL** and **cancer patient survival** [79–82].

"**Consistent with radiological observations of central necrosis in metastatic tumor nodules following DeltaRex-G treatment**, these histological observations of apoptosis, necrosis, and fibrosis within the tumor nodules are remarkably similar to those observed in preclinical studies, along with the observations of tumor infiltrating lymphocytes, as seen in the residual liver tumors of this biopsied liver. The appearance of immunoreactive T and B lymphocytes infiltrating from the normal hepatic tissues into the areas of tumor destruction in the residual liver tumors indicates that DeltaRex-G does not itself suppress or preclude local reactive immune responses" [17].

"**Among the classic hallmarks of DeltaRex-G action** — apoptosis, focal necrosis, anti-angiogenesis, immune cell infiltration, and reparative fibrosis ... [documenting patient immune activities:] ... CD+ leukocytes, helper-T and killer-T cells within the tumorous stroma, the latter of which tend to portend an improved overall survival" [59].

The Restored Immune Activities observed medically and histologically following repeated **DeltaRex-G** infusions involve cellular recognition and phagocytic removal of localized tumor debris [17–19]. Moreover, the *immune cell surges and resurgences* are evidently an active quantifiable component of the anti-cancer bioactivities of DeltaRex-G (*that is, the documented immunological, anti-angiogenic, phagocytic, and cancer cell-killing bioactivities*), which serve to reduce the viability of a **Flagrant Metastatic Tumor Nodule, as we espy in Figure 4**, to a few scant-clusters of cancer cells, shown here literally and figuratively *dying-on-the-vine* (**Figure 7**), and viewed histologically/microscopically amid overtly *swarming masses* of newly-recruited, identifiable immunological characters, which serve as a *Mobile* and *Rescuing* **Cavalry of Immune Cells** which arrive in support of the **dnG1-wielding Sheriffs**.

Because DeltaRex-G is the first *Lesion-Hunting/Cancer-Surveilling* Gene Therapy vehicle of its kind in history, this potentially "disruptive biotechnology exhibition" (aka *showdown*) —officially an "Investigational New Drug" (IND) with the U.S. FDA— was bound to be so thoroughly medically, socially, and scientifically scrutinized from the outset (including two formal NIH "RAC" reviews); so painstakingly *escalated to effective dose levels in the clinical setting*; so broadly challenged with a diverse menagerie of otherwise intractable chemotherapy-resistant cancers; and so judiciously handicapped as to proceed nonetheless with each allowable step in concert with the U.S. FDA—and yet, *oh,* so *cautiously* (investigationally) as salvage therapy, in the face of end-stage disease as a most brutal a testing ground! By demonstrating **(i) clinical safety (ii) single-agent efficacy, (iii) objective tumor responses, and (iv) survival benefits** in otherwise refractory metastatic cancers, the clinical utility of both the genetic payload (**dnG1** *killer gene*)

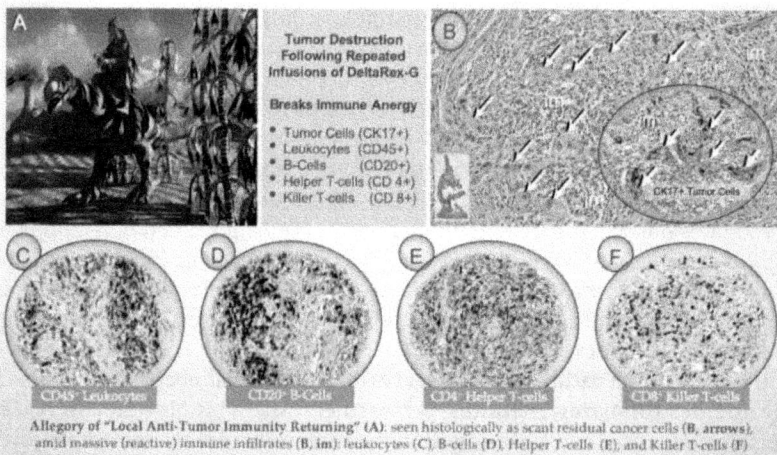

Figure 7.
Return of Innate Immune Responses following DeltaRex-G i.v. viewed histologically CLOSE-UP in pancreatic cancer. Elaborating the "Allegory of Restoration" (A) with Telltale Histology (B-F) as seen under a microscope. Far from a flagrant aggressive tumor, the scant remaining proliferative (CK17+) tumor cells (B) appear as being physically accosted by a veritable host of CD45+ leukocytes (C), which can be further sorted into CD20+ B-cells (D), CD4+ Helper T-cells (E), and CD8+ Killer T-cells (F) involved in the formation of "reactive" humoral (antibody-mediated) and Killer T-cell (cell-mediated) anti-tumor immunities, respectively, following repeated infusions of DeltaRex-G. Compare the apparent "nonresponsiveness" of (anergic, suppressed) immune reactivity surrounding the flagrant and robust **Outlaw pancreatic cancer cell formations** *seen in* **Figure 6,** *with the surrounded/dying corpses of the few remaining "CK-17+" (cytokeratin-positive) "Outlaw" Pancreatic Cancer Cells shown here, in this post-treatment-biopsy followed by immunohistochemical analysis, as mere remnants (B) surrounded by a gathering posse of immune response characters which tend to portend a favorable clinical outcome to treatment.*

and the tumor-targeting platform *(Nano-Dino-Hunting)* have been scientifically and medically validated ... well beyond dismissive contestation.

Restored contemporaneously with the *uniquely-American* **Right-To-Try legislation**: the advent of **Pathotropic Targeting** (aka proactive tumor-targeting) in clinical oncology—first embodied by **Rexin-G**, and faithfully restored (genetically, CMC; procedurally, cGMP) as **Delta-Rex-G (see Section 6)**—enables postmodern cancer patients and their clinical oncologists to reach beyond the field of the most gifted surgeon, beyond the reach of the finest catheters, to the very fabric of nature in relation to cancerous disease; to meet and safely match a formidable tumor burden, to enable more-effective clinical control of cancer metastasis, and to encourage the patient's natural (restored) immune responses to work in concert and harmony with the targeted gene therapy and the post-modern clinicians, respectively, in achieving such late-stage remissions [19, 77, 78].

6. Molecular mechanisms of a *Silver Bullet* revealed in action-adventure

Breaking Oncogene Addiction, Harnessing Cell-Competence, Restoring Law & Order.

With attention to **Bio-Pharmaceutical Safety,** as well as **Clinical Efficacy,** infusions of **DeltaRex-G** were proposed, reviewed, analyzed, and formally authorized by the U.S. FDA (and the Western Institution Review Board, WIRB). At each cautionary/pioneering stage of clinical development [15–22], a gradual, prudent, progressive **"Escalation of DeltaRex-G Infusions"** to higher **"Dose levels"** (tumor-targeted nanoparticles in Units/ml)—at one point, enabling a decisive (unprecedented) **"Across-the-Board" dose-escalation,** involving multiple ongoing clinical trials, following from quantitative statistical interim analyses and determinations of *Significant Survival Benefits,* first achieved in previously-intractable chemotherapy-resistant osteosarcomas and soft tissue sarcomas [78, 79], and subsequently achieved in clinical trials designed to include Stage 4 pancreatic cancer and many other types of *advanced* solid tumors [76–83].

Evaluation of the broad-spectrum Anti-cancer *Efficacy* of DeltaRex-G infusions from the benefit of patient history as well as histopathology is encouraging: Indeed, serious appreciation of such unprecedented *long-term cancer-free patient survival outcomes* encourages a good hard analytical squint at the actual "Smoking Gun" —the dnG1 *killer gene* **construct**— which was strategically (*i.e., biochemically genetically and structurally*) designed *expressly* for clinical oncology applications by Hall & Gordon [20, 83]. In terms of molecular and cellular biology, **the dnG1** *killer gene* is purposefully designed to disrupt an essential executive cell cycle control pathway (specific enzyme activity) governing "Mitotic Competence" (see **Figure 8**), thereby *Blocking* the G_0-to-G_1 (*Growth* phase transition) of normal reparative stem cells (*i.e., tumor cell accomplices*) and *Arresting* the uncontrolled proliferation of *genetically 'transformed' (Outlaw) Cancer Cells,* respectively. The main oncogenic i.e., "mechanistic drivers" of this **Commanding Cyclin G1/ Cdk/c-Myc/Mdm2**[(Hdm2)]**/p53 Axis** represent the enabling **"oncogene addictions"** and resulting **"genetic instabilities"** of a myriad of human cancer(s) [89, 90]. The central importance of **CCNG1(Cyclin G1)** expression and **"Cell Survival"** function in **"Tumorigenesis"** is substantiated by its consistent and persistent dysregulation in human cancers: Aberrantly elevated *CCNG1*(Cyclin G1) expression is associated with tumorigenesis, disease progression, EMT, metastasis, and chemotherapy resistance [20, 91–98]. Conversely, experimental blockade of *CCNG1*(Cyclin G1) expression in cancer cells by molecular-genetic approaches, including inhibitory microRNAs (e.g., miR-122, miR-27b, miR23b), confirms that functional blockade of *CCNG1*(Cyclin G1)-dependent pathways inhibits tumor growth, EMT, and metastasis, by functionally restoring sudden-death by Apoptosis in *(Outlaw)* **Cancer Cells** with the targeted (and enforced) expression of the **dnG1** *killer gene*, while sensitizing refractory tumor cells to chemotherapies [97–102].

In the language of cancer stem cell biology, thus future clinical oncology: loss or inactivation of normal p53 *tumor suppressor function* by genetic loss, inactivating mutation, or biochemical downregulation of the fragile *TP53 tumor suppressor* gene locus is mechanistically linked to high-grade cancers, tumorigenesis, and disease progression through the concomitant expression of the *CCNG1* (CyclinG1) **oncogene** [103]; elevated levels of the Cyclin G1 oncoprotein, often associated with a poor prognosis, drives an expanding self-renewing population of chemo-resistant *(Outlaw)* **Cancer Stem Cells** dangerously **Off-Road** [104]. Conversely, the restored or "enforced suppression" of the pivotal, driving *CCNG1/* Cyclin G1 oncogene overexpression by specific **CCNG1-gene-suppressive microRNAs (miRNAs)** prompts a remarkable biochemical "return-to-dormancy" in *stem-cell-like* liver cancer cells [105]. The central/pivotal importance of the **Cyclin G1 oncoprotein**, encoded by the *CYCG1 proto-oncogene* [106, 107], in governing cancer cell survival, competence, growth, and proliferation [108]—specifically, its *Executive Role* **in governing the Commanding Cyclin G1/c-Myc/ Mdm2**$^{(Hdm2)}$**/p53 Axis** [20, 83]—is presented diagrammatically in **Figure 8A**, representing the central biochemical underpinnings of **CANCER CELL**

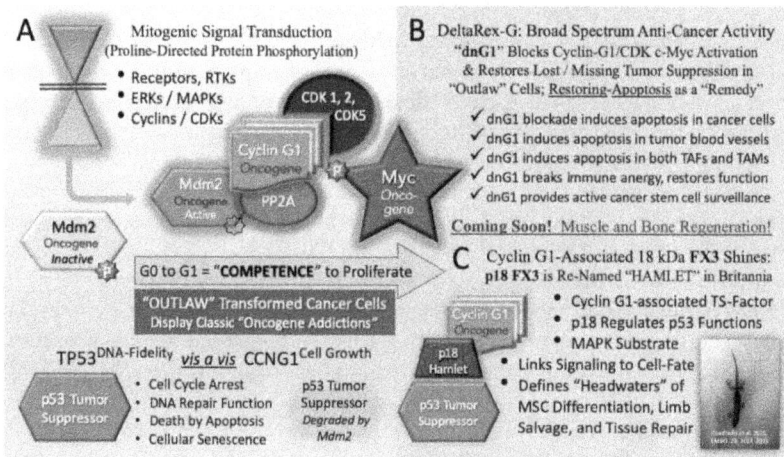

Figure 8.
*Science & Medicine on Sunset Blvd: Ushering "COMPETENCE" to clinical light. Hall and Gordon ultimately focused on blocking the **CCNG1/Cyclin G1** oncogene, an essential Survival Factor, which 'interfaces' with the TP53 Tumor Suppressor, and yet maintains Cyclin G1-dependent **Cell Viability over p53-mediated Perfection,** (DNA-fidelity) in the process of neoplastic transformation, and the face of (perverse) oncogene addiction(s), whereby the **Outlaw Cancer Stem Cells** remain, in a word: "HYPER-COMPETENT" to hide, to thrive opportunistically, and to proliferate flagrantly. The core oncogene-addicted card-players of "**Cancer Cell Competence**" are shown (in **Panel A**), as is the degradation of TP53/p53 by the Cyclin-G1 directed action of the MDM2/Hdm2 ubiquitin ligase. In the absence of natural p53 tumor suppression, **CCNG1/Cyclin G1** oncoprotein drives a sustained state of **Cell Competence** as observed in Cancer Stem Cells. By delivering the **dnG1** killer gene expression construct precisely to metastatic lesions (**Panel B**), DeltaRex-G unleashes a **Lethal Inhibitor of the Cyclin G1 Pathway,** which restores (the lost) **Tumor Suppression — Bang/Down! via Apoptosis!** Further studies of Cyclin G1/CDK-associated growth control pathways by Hall et al. in pediatric osteosarcomas (Children's Hospital Los Angeles) led to the identification and molecular cloning of **p18/FX3/Hamlet** by Fan Xu [84], a Cyclin-G1-associated Transcription Factor which interacts and cooperates with the TP53/p53 tumor suppressor—the natural Genome Guardian/Executioner of cellular **Bad Actors** [85–88]—to ensure the orderly differentiation of mesenchymal stem cells in a process called myogenesis, which governs **Cell Competence and DNA Fidelity** at the onset of **limb regeneration and tissue repair** (see Panel C).*

COMPETENCE: that is, the biochemical capability to grow, to replicate its genetic material, and to physically divide (mitosis). The clinical importance of this functional *cluster of key oncogenes* becomes clear when one considers the huge numbers of **'Advanced Metastatic Cancers'** that fit this *Outlaw Stem Cell profile*. Considering the broad-spectrum, single-agent efficacy observed with DeltaRex-G, in the context of long-term-cancer-free survivals: one can safely assume that DeltaRex-G—i.e., the Deputized Nano-Dino-*Sheriff* packing the **dnG1** *killer gene*—applied judiciously, repeatedly over sufficient time (in *Tumor-hunting-killing* pulses, no less)—brings a semblance of **Law & Order** to **flagrant** *Outlaws*: including notorious *Cancer Stem Cells and* their tumorigenic *Accomplices* (see **Figure 8B**).

Conceptually, mitogenic signal transduction cascades emanating from external stimulus: specifically from extracellular *growth-factor recepto*r*-mediated signaling events* that proceed ultimately through *"Proline-directed Protein Phosphorylation"* a major (digital) cell-regulatory theme: [109, 110], which can be divided enzymatically into **Mitogen-activated (extracellular signaling) protein kinases (MAPKs/ERKs)** [111–113] and **Cyclin-dependent protein kinase (CDK)** complexes that *govern* (control) the progressive phases of the animal cell division cycle. **CDKs** are a family of heterodimeric serine/threonine protein kinases: high-energy-phosphate-hurling enzymes, whose "physical activation" requires the *induction* (gene activation) hence *expression* of a relatively-unstable, often-oscillating **CDK-binding/molecular-targeting proteins**, called "Cyclins" [114]. Certain activating/targeting Cyclins are potential *oncogenes*, encoding a transforming *Cyclin oncoprotein,* which physically escorts its *otherwise* (clueless) *blind and inactive* cognate **CDK partner** [114, 115] to an executive molecular biological locus regulating *downstream* gene expression—hence exerting "**Executive Control**" of cell cycle progression [20, 83, 116]. Guided by fundamental understandings of chemical co-carcinogenesis: that is, seminal concepts of *Tumor Initiation* (i.e., DNA-damage) and *Tumor Promotion* (aberrant PKC enzymology), as observed in evolutionarily simple animal models of cancer [117, 118], we can now affirm with hard-core molecular mechanisms and museum-quality science [118], *malignant reticuloma of the lowly planarian resides in the **Smithsonian** archives*], which declares that **Cancer is** *— first and foremost —* a Stem Cell Disease.

A Brief Reflection on the Prospects of Wound Healing, Limb Salvage, Spinal Regeneration:

"**To-Be**"**or** "**Not-to-Be?!**" Following the identification, molecular cloning, and functional characterization of the human *CYCG1/CCNG1* (Cyclin G1) oncogene [106–108] by Hall et al. at Children's Hospital Los Angeles, Hall's laboratory identified several "*associated*" human genes, including a *Zinc-finger-containing* protein, **p18**[FX3], originally isolated in a molecular two-hybrid screen for human "*Cyclin-G1-associated* proteins" [84]; This **p18/FX3** gene was recently re-discovered and aptly re-named **p18/Hamlet** — "*based on its ability to control life-or-death cell-fate decisions*" [85]. Such *fateful* cellular decisions are determined mechanistically by a veritable cascade of signal transductions, linking the p38-α mitogen-activated protein kinase (MAPK14) to the *Guardian/Executioner* (apoptosis) functions of the **p53** *tumor suppressor* protein through a direct biochemical association with the **Cyclin G1** *oncoprotein* (**Figure 8C**). The curious **p18/Hamlet** protein was determined to participate in *cell cycle arrest* in response to DNA-damaging agents by acting cooperatively as a (transcriptional co-activator) with the **p53** *tumor suppressor* **protein** [86], inducing *Apoptosis* in proliferative stem cells, *aka blast cells*, by selectively activating the "promoter regions" of pro-apoptotic genes [87]. Histologically, **p18/Hamlet** protein levels are low in proliferating myoblasts; yet are upregulated during normal muscle differentiation, which correlates with phosphorylation (regulation) by p38/MAPK14 signal transduction cascades. In addition to providing an allegorically eloquent and clinically pertinent **biomarker of Cell Fate** for cancer stem cell profiling and treatment monitoring, **p18/Hamlet** is recruited in a p38/MAPK (phosphorylation)-dependent manner to the "myogenin" promoter at the onset of myogenesis and muscle differentiation [88]; thereby, linking extracellular signal transduction to gene expression, cell proliferation, and DNA-fidelity through the decisive executive enzymology of cellular growth control. Much like a "**Western Showdown**" at the *Crossroads* of cell proliferation, muscle differentiation, and tissue regeneration: this **Cyclin-G1-*associated***, nuclear-targeted **p18/Hamlet** protein binds to the **p53** tumor suppressor to help *Enforce* the Apoptosis of aberrant cells. Developmentally, the intrinsic regulation of this **Commanding Cyclin G1/Cdk/c-Myc/Mdm2$^{(Hdm2)}$/p53 Axis** functions as a pivotal biochemical *fulcrum* whereby protein **Survival Factors** and **Tumor Suppressors** "**engage and interact biochemically thus cooperatively**" in regulating genomic stability in the somatic cells (that is, bodily cells) of *all multicellular animals* [119].

Biochemically speaking, the decisive CCNG1/Cyclin G1 oncoprotein, along with its cognate **Cyclin-dependent kinase (Cdk) partner**, physically "Activates" (by site-specific protein phosphorylation) the **c-Myc oncoprotein** — the evanescent and indisputable "*Star*" of "*Cell COMPETENCE*" (see **Figures 8** and **9**) [121–128]. Beyond demonstrations, proofs, and teachings that *Cyclin G1 blockade is a rational, strategic locus for precision cancer gene therapy* [20, 78, 83], this applied pharmacological "*Blockade of c-Myc Activation*" is of major clinical importance — c-Myc "*Activation*" *of growth control genes regulating cell cycle progression* has long been considered to be the "*most desirable locus*" and yet the "*least druggable target*" in all of cancer therapy [121–126]. Thus, by activating/ stabilizing c-Myc gene regulatory function, the *CCNG1 (Cyclin G1)* **governs the** *first-and-rate-limiting step* in the executive control of animal cell proliferation. From the perspective of **precision Cancer Gene Therapy**, the cytocidal dominant-negative **dnG1** *expression construct* "**Arrests**" mitotic cell division cycle and thereby "**reEnforces**" the weakened/lost tumor suppressor, executioner, apoptosis functions of *TP53(p53)*, which is commonly (tragically) lost with the development, spread, and clinical progression of metastatic cancers. The central importance of aberrant *CCNG1*/Cyclin G1 expression as a "*Biochemical Driver*" of oncogenic transformation is supported by the demonstrated clinical anticancer activity of the **dnG1 killer gene construct** [20, 83]. **Clinically** *[as Precision Cancer Gene Therapy]*, enforced expression of the **dnG1** *killer gene construct* in proliferative animal cells is uniformly lethal; even in genetically damaged, oncogene-addicted, rapidly-evolving, chemotherapy-resistant, hyper-competent cancer cells; that is, advanced *Metastatic Cancers* derived from **any of the** *three primitive germ layers* of our developmental embryology (skin, bone, glands); thereby re-enforcing/ restoring '**Tumor Cell Death by Apoptosis**' and eliminating a host of cellular *Bad Actors* — including and especially *nasty Cancer Stem Cells* — with tumor-targeted therapeutic gene delivery. In terms of the **Clinical Oncology**: there is a proverbial "*New Sheriff in Town*" — the **DeltaRex-G** *gene vector* — capable of delivering the **dnG1** *silver bullets (to an operating theater near you)* with biochemical precision.

From the perspective of **cancer research**, intrinsic tumor suppressive mechanisms evolved naturally in multicellular animals, and most necessarily in long-lived and/or large-size mammals, including humans, elephants, and sperm whales—each embodying increasing populations of renewable stem cells, which remain constantly vulnerable to perilous oncogenic mutations. Potent *tumor suppressive mechanisms* were acquired to maintain both genetic stability and the appropriate numbers of cells within tissues; additionally, stem cell activation, cell division, death, and survival are tightly regulated by *social cues*, including growth factor stimulation, attachment to collagenous basement membranes, contact with other

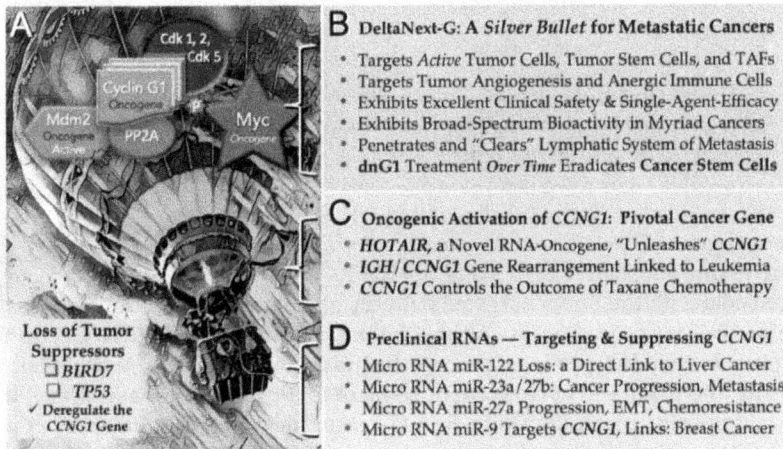

Figure 9.
Cyclin-G1/c-Myc 'COMPETENCE' Rising with the Loss of Tumor Suppressors. (A) The Cyclin G1/c-Myc/ Mdm2(Hdm2)/p53 Axis of Cancer Cell COMPETENCE depicted here as a rising assembly of oncogenes wherein the Loss of Tumor Suppression, in the form of BIRD7 and/or TP53, reveals a central and ascending role of the CCNG1/CyclinG1 oncogene. (B) Objective clinical, radiological, histological, cytological evidence of anti-tumor/anti-cancer activity is observed with DeltaNext-G, dominant negative (dnG1) Cyclin G1 knockout construct. (C) Hot New Discoveries, including the novel RNA-Oncogene HOTAIR, and a tragic genetic (presumably iatrogenic) breakpoint translocation IGH/CCNG1, which may lead to leukemias in cancer chemotherapy patients—affirm the Cyclin G1 oncogene as a strategic target for cancer therapy. (D) Likewise, a conclave of new regulatory/gene-suppressive microRNA species have been discovered, which (i) are lost with stem cell transformation and progression to cancer, (ii) are directly linked to elevated CCNG1/ Cyclin G1 expression, and (iii) thus represent future gene-regulatory/therapy medicines [120]—pending translational research and eventual development of safe, effective clinical-stage therapeutic/oncogene-suppressive microRNA delivery systems.

somatic cells, and with adequate blood supply [129]. In studying the elephant, we find that the biochemical modality of intrinsic tumor suppression is focused on the evolution of multiple copies of the TP53 gene (i.e., gene dosage) yielding an appreciable increase in sensitivity and responsiveness to DNA damage involving *TP53* (p53) expression, forms, and functions [130, 131]. While it is generally known that mutational loss and/or inactivation of the **TP53 locus**, observed in ≥50% of human cancers, is a major downhill road that leads to tumorigenesis in humans [132]; it was only recently reported in ovarian cancer that a mutation of TP53 leads rather directly to the dysregulation of **CCNG1 (Cyclin G1)** expression, which thereby promotes the high-grade cancer, EMT, tumorigenesis, chemotherapy resistance, and disease progression [103]. As shown in **Figure 9**, DeltaRex-G represents a potential *Silver Bullet for metastatic cancers*—delivered actively and selectively to primary and metastatic lesions, the **dnG1** *killer gene*, a *Blocking construct*, counteracts Cyclin G1/CDK dependent-pathways, thus the *Outlaw* behavior of cancer cells.

7. Raising the bar for *metastatic cancer survival and quality-of-life*

Long-Term Cancer-Free Survival: A New "Gold-Standard" for Objective Responses.

In reviewing our progress, dear reader, we have traveled *Far-Off-Road*, into the uncharted landscapes of metastatic cancers, traveling into a bewildering state of **Collagenous Anaplasia**, explored, documented, and **Mapped-out histologically** with proactive Pathotropic tumor-targeting:

I. **By a *Nano-Dino-Hunting* Metastasis** — via repeated intravenous infusions of DeltaRex-G.

II. **By Delivering a Molecular *"Silver Bullet"* — dnG1, a broad-spectrum killer gene aimed at disrupting Cancer Cell Competence-to-Proliferate** (depicted graphically in **Figures 8** and **9**).

Conceptually, the Cyclin G1-dependent "**Activation**" of the **c-Myc protooncogene** [126–128] is simply *out-of-control* in transformed, oncogene-addicted (*Outlaw*) cancer cells; while aberrant *Outlaw stem cell "activation"* is stopped cold with the tumor-targeted delivery of **DeltaRex-G**, administered safely and effectively as monotherapy. Although the **non-canonical CCNG1/Cyclin G1 oncoprotein remains, perhaps, among the most mysterious and *least understood* of all the executive cell cycle control elements** [20, 133–136], the inescapable clinical conclusion regarding **Delta-Rex-G** cancer therapy is this: *Blockade of Cyclin G1 function by physiological tumor-targeting (i.e., proactive cancer sur-veillance) with enforced dnG1 gene expression* is broadly effective as an anti-cancer agent [20], thereby providing objective clinical responses and survival benefits, even in prior end-stage chemotherapy-resistant metastatic cancer patients [76–83].

Evaluating clinical cancer surveillance and precision anti-cancer activity of **DeltaRex-G:** The Pathotropic (tumor-targeted) gene delivery vehicle, **DeltaRex-G**, performs sufficiently-well in *"Hunting-Tracking Metastatic Cancers Off-Road"* amid daunting physiological barriers, shear forces, turbulence, filtrations, dilutions, and blood flows of the human systemic circulation, including metastatic oozes and cancerous disseminations into the lymphatic drainage [137]; *"Hunting"* sufficiently-well, that is, to reach, penetrate, alter disease processes, and eventually eradicate the *totality* of previously intractable metastatic disease, as in the first documented cases of long-term cancer-free survival [17–22, 81–83], as updated (in accord with FDA guidance) with interim analysis and case reports documenting prior and ongoing clinical trials [138–141]. Given sufficient daily/ weekly doses of DeltaRex-G —with intent to approach and safely reach a mathe-matical '*Parity*' (equivalence) with the flagrant and growing '*Tumor Burden*'— **long-term survival, *carefully managed*, now appears to be an achievable clinical goal** [22].

Determined by regulatory authorities to be **Exceptionally Safe**, by virtue of (i) DeltaRex-G design features and vector engineering, (ii) progressive dose-escalation studies, and (iii) insightful clinical experiences reaching beyond *salvage therapy* into *hospice care* (under **Compassionate Use protocols**), the documented **Objec-tive Clinical Responses to DeltaRex-G** in the course of treating of Stage 4 meta-static disease, includes overt anti-angiogenesis and altered immune infiltrations, with concomitant focal necrosis and cellular apoptosis observed in all classes of flagrant proliferative tumor cells—accomplishing complete eradication of prior chemotherapy-resistant primary and secondary metastatic lesions. The clinical doc-umentation of progression-free survival, overall survival, and long-term cancer-free survival in a growing number of otherwise intractable chemotherapy-resistant cancers—along with the overt histology of phagocytic immune activation (innate immune activities) with infiltrations of B- and T-lymphocytes—**suggests the participation of a 'restored' adaptive (acquired) antitumor immunity** [17–22, 76–83]. Indeed, further-analysis of tumor biopsies obtained from a variety of such long-term survivors reveals positive enhancement of immune cell trafficking in the tumor microenvironment of advanced-stage DeltaRex-G/dnG1-treated cancers is a consistent cytological feature:

> *"This underscores the advantageous pleotropic effects of DeltaRex-G: killing tumor cells, and conceivably promoting cancer immunization in situ"* [142].

WANTED: All Dead and Gone! Wanted—each and every DNA-damaged, genetically transformed, fiercely-independent, human genome-possessing, **CCNG1 (Cyclin-G1)-expressing**, oncogene-addicted, CTHRC1-wielding, *Outlaw* **Cancer Cell** that is rapidly EMT transitioning, aggressively metastasizing into the gristly *Anaplastic Territories* of the histological *Inner Dark*; cancer cells "jail-breaking" out of growth constraining collagenous cages, taking innocent cells hostage, immune-suppressing, biochemically evading detection, migrating lymphatically [137], waiting-out the ravaging storms of ineffectual apothecary (cytotoxic chemotherapy), hiding-out in every histological *hole in the wall* with clinical manifestations of disseminated metastatic disease. Alas, when standard chemotherapy-inevitably fails to control badass metastatic cancers, like pancreatic cancer, for example [143], **so-called CANCER STEM CELLS re-EMERGE, even now *More-Aggressive* and profoundly CHEMORESISTANT!!** By the time cancer Stage 4 cancer patents *qualified* to receive tumor-targeted DeltaRex-G (i.e., **dnG1 *silver bullets***) as monotherapy, under previous FDA approved rules of engagement, Hall & Gordon et al., were often faced with clinical cases presenting horrific (quantitative) tumor burdens, often described radiologically in PET/CT scans as *"too many tumors to count!!"*

It is in this dire context: In the context of chemotherapy resistance, in the context of widespread cancer metastasis, in the face of overwhelming physiological obstacles, tumor burdens, risk/benefit ratios, and life-support considerations, that (i) profound demonstrations of single agent efficacy, (ii) documentation of actual tumor-targeting, (iii) characterization of restored anti-tumor immune responses, and (iv) the elimination of cancer stem cells have been achieved pharmacologically. **It is in this dire context** that metastatic tumor-eradication, progression-free-survival, and long-term-survival have been achieved clinically—with infusions of **DeltaRex-G** delivering **dnG1 *silver bullets*** in the mean streets of cancer metastasis, in the crucible of clinical oncology. Importantly, these tumor-busting gene therapy *bullets* are delivered by a discerning "safety-minded" Sheriff: a **synthetic vector** that only *"shoots"* and *"kills"* *proliferative* tumor cells, guided by a proactive Pathotropic *(lesion seeking)* Nano-Dino-Hunter, which can be delivered intravenously, safely and repeatedly, in therapeutic pulses, in an effort to meet and match an unrestrained tumor burden.

Targeted Gene Delivery!
What was once the elusive *"Holy Grail"* of card-carrying gene therapists ...
Tumor Anti-angiogenesis!
What was once the illustrious *"Battle*-Cry" of Dr. Folkman's War on cancer ...
The c-Myc proto-Oncogene and Oncogene Addiction!!
What was once lamented as an *undruggable* aspect of oncogenic transformation ...
Chemotherapy Resistance! and Multidrug Resistance!
What was once considered a confounding property of *Outlaw* Cancer Cell behavior; often considered adequate explanation for multiple therapeutic failures...
Intractable *Outlaw* Cancer Stem Cells!
What was once considered an insurmountable problem of cancer recurrence.

Historically, and herein dramatically in reference to the epic "STANDOFF" of critical oncological aims and opinions displayed above, we present a clinical/medical "SHOWDOWN" —a quaint, albeit iconic, demonstration of Wild-West daring-do—starring **DeltaRex-G, a precision-guided nanotechnological Sheriff** (*Law and Order*) function, which simply does what it was purposefully designed to do: **To**

deliver Biologic Therapy (dnG1 *silver bullets*) precisely into *Outlaw* **Cancer Cells** and their intimidated **tumor-cell accomplices** found lurking/hiding acting ruthlessly within the cancerous/metastatic "**Inner Dark**" of diseased tissues. Herein we present a Western-style SHOWDOWN wherein lofty clinical aims like *single-agent efficacy, broad-spectrum activity, dose dependent efficacy, metastatic tumor eradication, and long-term cancer survival* come face-to-face with entrenched, obstinate, and outdated opinions concerning the limits and utility of toxic chemotherapies *vis-a-vis* the objective realities of measured things, including patient lifetimes .... .

Surely, all of these professional, medical, explanatory, yet abating "**Opinions of Things**" will now have to be reconsidered in light of long-term Cancer-free Survival and Quality of Life (QOL) improvements presently achieved & documented in a growing number of otherwise intractable cancers, with repeated pulsed *i.v.* infusions of tumor-targeted **DeltaRex-G**—*given in sufficient quantities*, and *over an extended treatment-period of time*. Following the logic: if and when a Stage 4 metastatic cancer patient is (1) relieved of tumor burden and (2) determined to be cancer-free for greater than 10 years—with no additional treatments, as documented with DeltaRex-G patients over the past two decades—both scientists and clinicians can eventually agree: regardless of historic positions and opinions on the matter ... that the *Cancer Stem Cell Culprits* were indeed "caught-up" and included in the *precision-targeted* **dnG1 Shootout**! Evidently, **DeltaRex-G** *hunts-down* metastatic cancers, as designed, and delivers the **dnG1** *killer gene* efficiently into tumors: including the notorious, chemotherapy-resistant *Outlaw* **Cancer Stem Cells** that are *hiding out* (presumably from the chemotherapy) in the protective quasi-dormancy of metastatic tumors. As a further intellectual exercise in evaluating contemporary cancer therapies, compare: (i) the relentless *Slope(s)* to "**Zero**" *of the dismal "Survival Curves"* following standard approved chemotherapies for pancreatic cancer, as aggregated and tallied in the current medical literature [143] versus (ii) the observable, repeatable, thus achievable *dose-dependent improvements* in **Stage 4 metastatic cancer "Survival Times**," as documented with cited with references herein; as visualized photographically, graphically, and pictographically in **Figure 10**.

With the upward suspended "Harpoon" of Melville's Seagoing Captain still held metaphorically high ... (!) we hear an echo from voice of good counsel from the battlefields of our historic past:

> *"To heal him [rather them] you need to touch something.*
> *other [deeper] than the coverlet of his [their] bedsheets."*
>
> Ambroise Paré, ***Journeys in Diverse Places***, 1569.

As modern clinical oncology and much of pharmaceutical science simply throws up its figurative hands in collective despair over chemotherapeutic refractoriness, while chasing/profiling cancer-related red herrings (i.e., variable logically-vague tumor antigens) with abandon [68, 69], but alas, with little positive effects on **survival time**. Thus, we must *Focus Intensely* (biologically and intellectually) upon the troublesome and *disturbing* **CANCER STEM CELL**, as the leading *Badass Culprit* (*Outlaw* Cancer Cell) which apparently refuses to cooperate with chemotherapy; and yet these *Outlaw* **Cancer Stem Cells** "disappear" after cancer patients have achieved a sustained remission of unabated metastatic disease progression (to cancer-free status) with sufficient **Delta-Rex-G treatment**—gradually gaining control of the entire tumor burden. By providing a *Physiological Tumor Surveillance* which evidently kills residual Cancer Stem Cells over an extended period of time, DeltaRex-G appears to be aided perhaps by the observed and documented *Restoration of the Immune System*, which often accompanies clinical remission.

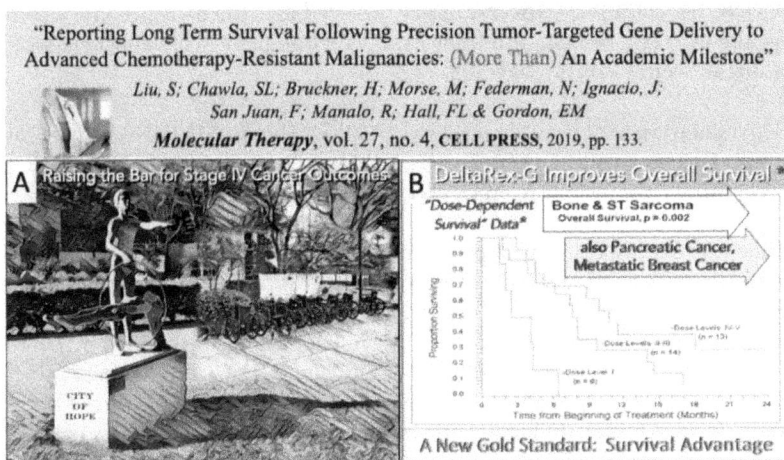

Figure 10.
Appreciable dose-dependent improvements in metastatic cancer survival times. Re-Examining and statistically raising the issue of "Time" at the extreme **hard right edge** *of cancer statistical survival graphs. (A) In 2019, the* Aveni-Mission to restore DeltaRex-G bioproduction site-visited the City of Hope, an NCI-designated comprehensive cancer center, where the A-Team met with officials and scientists at the **Center for Gene Therapy** *to discusses the unique needs for producing (cGMP) tumor-targeted medicines, and to advance the development new gene therapy options for metastatic cancer patients. (B) The Kaplan–Meier method is a graphic method of analyzing survival data where the response variable is the length of time taken to reach a certain end-point, often death, as shown above. The observed Dose-dependent efficacy physically* **Raises the Bar** *from the relentless certainty of patient death—as is shown graphically here at FDA-requested lowest-doses of DeltaRex-G—to appreciably longer-term survival at higher effective DeltaRex-G doses, as (i) the tumor burden is progressively reduced, (ii) immune responses are restored, (iii) Cancer Stem Cells are eliminated, and (iv) remissions are extended in time. On the "x-axis, marking* **Time from Beginning of Treatment,** *longer is better [144]; compare a recent "nationwide chart review" compiling dismal results of the major standard chemotherapies [143].*

Investigating the **Stem Cell Culprits**—lurking within the scary and life-threatening *neo-Noir* of the metastatic **"Inner Dark,"** we detect what Old-Time *Private Investigators* as well as conscientious physician-scientists refer to as **"Important Clues**: each one representing a complex molecular mechanism-of-action, yet presented here for expediency, simplicity, and dramatic impact as these **Six hard-core** *Silver Bullet* **points to consider**!!!!!!

1. **CCNG1Cyclin G1 expression** *per se*—via the **Cyclin G1/CDK/Mdm2/p53 Axis**—regulates drug sensitivity-to multiple cancer chemotherapeutic agents: including all the Taxanes, Doxorubicin, Vincristine, 5-Flurouracil, and cisplatinum [97–102].

2. **CCNG1(Cyclin G1) expression** *per se*—regulates the **Epithelial-to-Mesenchymal Transition** to an aggressively "metastatic" cell phenotype associated with disease progression [101, 145].

3. **The Cyclin G1**-dependent **CDK/Mdm2/p53 Axis** links the cellular phenomenon of **Epithelial-to-Mesenchymal Plasticity** to the intricate molecular mechanisms **Chemotherapy Resistance** [146].

4. **CCNG1(Cyclin G1)** *per se*—is officially ranked as a **Cancer Stem Cell** *"Marker"* based on genome-wide profiling for unique pertinent *pluripotent* i.e., *Stem Cell Signatures* [147].

5. **CCNG1(Cyclin G1) expression** *per se*—mediates the poor prognosis of **high-grade ovarian, breast, and liver cancers** through an *expanding population* of **Cancer Stem Cells** in [103–105, 147].

6. **Upregulation** of the survival-linked *CCNG1(CyclinG1)* 'stem cell gene' in multidrug resistant **Leukemia cells** reveals a *Drug Resistance Stem Cell program that is* switched-on *en bloc* [148].

While this manuscript was in preparation, in early 2020, we became aware by pre-publication of an exceedingly important medical paper concerning the **CCNG1 (Cyclin G1) proto-oncogene:** (*Haematologica, Volume 105; doi:10.3324/haema tol.2020.246744)*—wherein Harvard and Mayo Clinic investigators led by Dr. Sheng Xiao reported a novel genetic mutation, specifically **IGH-CCNG1 gene rearrangement,** that was found in a patient with *chemotherapy-induced* acute myeloid leukemia (AML). This specific mutation could therefore potentially serve as a target for therapeutic **DeltaRex-G** infusions as tumor-targeted gene therapy, for the *designer* **dnG1** *killer gene* construct is a proven **CCNG1 (Cyclin G1 pathway) inhibitor.**

According to Dr. Xiao et al., of Harvard University:

*"Clinical trials with a dominant-negative CCNG1 retroviral expression vector (DeltaRex-G) showed impressive results, including several metastatic tumors being cancer-free ten years after **DeltaRex-G monotherapy**.... It will be interesting to evaluate how frequent the CCNG1 is overexpressed in myeloid tumors, and whether an anti-CCNG1 strategy such as DeltaRex-G is effective in treating myeloid tumors, a group of diseases typically with very poor prognosis"* [149].

Consistent with these findings, Gordon and co-workers have shown that the *CCNG1* (Cyclin G1) gene is highly expressed in many cancer types and they are presently developing companion diagnostic assays to identify patients who are likely to benefit from **DeltaRex-G** treatment [150].

This striking discovery of an oncogenic breakpoint translocation at the **CCNG1 gene** *promoter* region is clinically and oncologically revealing: It affirms that the *overexpression of the Cyclin G1 oncoprotein is sufficient*—by itself (via Cyclin G1/Cdk Axis Hyper-activity)—*to actually Cause Cancer, in this case,* an acute and deadly myeloid leukemia.

Future investigations will necessarily include a fine-grain histopathological and molecular-genetic analysis of this hyperactive, oncogenic **Cyclin G1/CDK/c-Myc/Mdm2**[(Hdm2)] **Axis,** which favors cell survival, *sans* TP53 (see **Figures 8** and **9**):

i. to improve differential diagnosis and cancer staging with *Pertinent Biomarkers.*

ii. to determine the extent to which *Restored Immune Responses* versus *Cancer Stem Cell removal* (via **dnG1** *silver bullets*) best characterize the objective responses and histological eradications of flagrant tumors observed following repeated intravenous infusions of the **dnG1** *killer gene* delivered proactively to tumors as **DeltaRex-G.**

In a dramatic and climactic state of affairs such as this: Stage 4 Cancer, wherein, **Cancer Stem Cells, EMT, and Drug Resistance** can be envisioned conceptually as *"An Emerging Axis-of-Evil in the War on Cancer"* [151], then **DeltaRex-G** might well be envisioned as a **multi-tasking** *"Peacemaker,"* **in the vernacular of the Wild West**—delivering the **dnG1** *killer gene precisely,* as needed. At the end of the day, *you now have a legal Right-to-Know* this new biomedical information, thus an opportunity to consider real things like survival very carefully, as well as a *legal* **Right to Try**.

8. The success of a raindance depends a lot on timing (cowboy proverb)

Passing Fallacies, Failed Hypotheses, and a Cancer-Surveillance Platform Restored.

The demands of **Multicellularity**, like the demands of **Truth**, are severe. Whereas unicellular organisms (and viruses) parade *genetic instability* as a virtue in terms of survival and evolution, the fidelity of DNA-replication in the body of **a multicellular organism** (i.e., *over one's lifetime*) is of paramount importance, such that maintaining *genetic fidelity (that is, fidelity of DNA replication)* is how we manage to stay the same each day/week/month/year as human beings. The Genomic Stability of multicellular animal cells can be considered a matter of high-level top-down **Homeostasis**: A revered principle of life (and concept of medicine) which declares: *"The stability of the internal environment* [the milieu intérieur] *is the condition for the free and independent life."* All multicellular animals—including celebrated fruit flies, sea urchins, planarians, frogs, salamanders, mice, dogs, humans, elephants, and even the great whales—have the same **STEM CELL DNA-Fidelity Issues** and the same conserved molecular-genetic mechanisms linking *Cell-Life* and *Cell-Death Decisions* to the hard core biochemistries governing **Stem Cell Competence: competence** to respond to external cues: competence to become activated *en-bloc* in terms of gene expression, competence to grow larger, followed by fastidious/exacting **DNA-replication (of its genome)**, followed by the elaborate processes of chromosome re-distribution and actual **stem cell division** [20, 83].

Having traveled back in evolutionary time (with biomedical research) to pierce the very fabric of nature and metastatic disease, scientists can now declare with molecular-genetic certainty that "**TP53 and CCNG1(Cyclin G1) do indeed cooperate in mediating genome stability in somatic animal cells**" [119]. Having identified the **TP53 (p53)** tumor suppressor as the major prototypical *Guardian & Executioner* of genetically damaged cells, biochemists and medical oncologists can and do declare with some molecular-genetic certainty that (**see Figures 8** and **9**): "*All the roads* **involving functional mutations in TS53(p53) lead to tumorigenesis**" [129–132]. Moreover, it also appears clear that mutational loss or inactivation of the **TP53(p53)** *tumor suppressor* leads rather directly to *abnormal overexpression* of the **CCNG1(Cyclin G1) proto-oncogene**, a countervening *Survival factor*, which is subject to oncogene-addiction [89, 90], as well as viral-subversion [152], and is responsible for the metastatic progression of ovarian cancer [103], as well as the expansion of the populations of *Outlaw* **Cancer Stem Cells** which apparently mediate the poor prognosis of metastatic breast and liver cancer [104, 105].

Herein, we present a central unifying theme in the form of **The Pivotal and Commanding Cyclin G1/Cdk/c-Myc/HDM2/p53 Axis (20, 83)** – which defines and delimits the *hyper*-**Competent, oncogene-addicted, tumor suppressor-deficient** state of **all aggressive, EMT, migratory, i.e., metastatic human cancers** (**Figure 8**). We present this bold, reductionist, picturesque, view of the genetic profile of the notorious **Cancer Stem Cell**—main *Outlaw* **Character on Wild West WANTED Posters**—yet perhaps most importantly, we present this Pivotal Axis—*a profile of unbridled Oncogenes*—as a bulwark against a rising tide of molecular occultism, as seen in relation to superficial cancer profiling [68], as needed in relation to more seriously safe and effective anti-cancer therapies.

As we come to the end of this Good/Bad/Ugly rattlesnake roundup of scientific papers, medical publications, clinical reports, issued patents, FDA-approvals, and

Intellectual Property Badges, we find **"the Good"** in the broad-spectrum anti-cancer efficacy, safety, and survival value of the **dnG1** *silver bullet* in the face of intractable metastatic disease. We find **"the Bad"** in the telltale discovery of a newfound *chemotherapy-induced* acute myelogenous leukemia (AML) resulting from a genetic mutation at the *CCNG1*(Cyclin G1) gene promoter region, leading consequently to the aberrant overexpression of the Cyclin G1 oncoprotein, leading ontologically to a tragic case of AML [149]. The NEWS here is that **"the Good"** (**DeltaRex-G/dnG1** *silver bullet*) may indeed represent a new strategic treatment for AML, **"the** *chemotherapy-induced* **Bad."** Finally we find "the **Ugly**" in the *popularized* public branding & promotion of "buffered chemotherapies" presented mistakenly as cutting-edge *tumor-targeted* nanotechnologies [153], which led to formal FDA criticisms, scientific retractions [154–156], and **disappointing Survival Results in late stage clinical trials,** prompting the reputable clinical investigators to issue a notice of serious medical criticism at the disappointing conclusion of a large-scale comparative Phase III trial for locally recurrent or metastatic breast cancer:

> *"Without direct evidence, the earlier trials led to widespread use of more costly and higher-dose nab-paclitaxel in many clinical practices. The higher dose used in our Phase III trial resulted in early discontinuation and dose reductions, which in turn limited exposure to the drug. On the basis of our data, once-per-week paclitaxel should remain the preferred microtubule inhibitor for treating patients with metastatic Breast Cancer in the first-line setting, and there is no evidence that either of the newer agents is superior"* [157].

According to Lord Kelvin (aka William Thompson; eminent physicist, inventor), *"When you cannot express it in numbers, your understanding is of a very meager and unsatisfactory kind."* In other words, when the so-called treatments that are presently propounded don't add up to significant quantitative improvements in either *survival or quality of life*—you all got Zilch!

Another inexorable *critique* re the Good, the Bad, and the Ugly of modern-day cancer therapy—in terms of objective clinical truth *vis a vis* hand-waving contrivances, dubious petri-dish connivances, and *lowdown* biomedical thinking—is the perineal and yet pernicious bio-*pharmaceutical mindset* which carelessly, intentionally hurls **'live viruses'** at immune-compromised cancer patients with a-lick-and-a-promise, which tends to end badly. At this point (public *education*), it should suffice to mention yet-another major *clinical disappointment* in our contemporary times, wherein card-carrying armchair experts and key 'opinion leaders' in the emerging fields of cancer gene therapy & immunotherapy hawk tantalizing **"Demonstrations of therapeutic efficacy in an orthotopic immune-competent mouse glioma model"** (actual title) ... thereby proclaiming, *"On the basis of these and other supporting data, a clinical trial investigating intravenous administration of **Toca 511** in patients with recurrent HGG is currently open and enrolling."* [158, 159]; only to finally admit complete failure (*no endpoints met*) by the end of the day [160, 161] – thus terminating the clinical fiasco, but not the end of the appropriate scientific criticisms. Apparently, the chronicles of non-targeted agents, live infectious viruses, and/or untethered immunological cancer therapies are sufficiently dismal in these present times to re-examine the entire approach from a scientific point of view: judging from the title, content, and the *calling cards* of the seven distinguished authors reporting on the *First Annual Remission Summit* [162]: (In Press, May 2020).

> **"Adult Immuno-Oncology: Using Past Failures to Inform the Future.**
> *In this context, the past, present and future of immune-oncology for the treatment of glioblastoma GBM was discussed by clinical, research and thought leaders as well as*

> patient advocates at the first annual Remission Summit in 2019. The goal was to use
> current knowledge (published and unpublished) to identify possible causes of
> treatment failures and the best strategies to advance immunotherapy as a
> treatment modality for patients with GBM. The discussion focuses on past
> failures, current limitations, failure analyses and proposed best practices moving
> forward."

In light of our combined 40 years of hunting metastatic cancers with tumor-targeted gene therapy vectors, we applaud this enlightened social criticism. In view of our guiding philosophies and objective clinical experiences with precision-guided, replication-incompetent, pro-active (Pathotropic) disease-seeking gene vectors, including DeltaRex-G and Reximmune-C, we simply reiterate our principled position:

> **"Caution! A Modern Medicine Should Not a Replicating Species Be**
> *At this point, a categorical distinction—indeed, a moral distinction—must be made
> between the replication incompetent retroviral vector (presented herein), which is
> constructed from inert components with no replication competent characteristics,
> and the infectious species of viruses that has been advocated in recent years with
> a disturbing epidemiological naiveté and a less-than-convincing scientific rationale"*
> [78].

The use of the **"C"-word**, as in *"Cured of advanced chemotherapy-resistant metastatic cancers,"* is still fraught with contentious implications for patients and physicians, as well as a concerned society [163, 164]; thus, necessitating the restrained announcement of *an Academic Milestone* (see **Figure 10**). In all seriousness, the privilege of observing long-standing **DeltaRex-G**-induced clinical remissions and long-term cancer-free survival surpassing 10-Years running, in cases of previously intractable chemotherapy resistant pancreatic cancer, osteosarcoma, breast cancer, and soft tissue sarcoma [20, 22, 82, 83, 138–142]—is an epic achievement which everyone can celebrate.

Future clinical studies will focus on determining *when* and *to what extent* **Restoration of the Immune System**, as visualized in **Figure 7**, versus *Outlaw* **Cancer Stem Cell Control**, as elaborated in **Figures 8** and **9**, serves descriptively to eradicate stubborn chemotherapy-resistant malignancies. Future clinical studies will also address issues of **"Fibroblast Activation"** and *Outlaw* **Cancer Cell** *"Hostage-Taking"* on a molecular level, as local fibroblasts (innocent bystanders) are reprogrammed biochemically by *Outlaw* Cancer Cells to become tumorigenic accomplices, i.e., cancer-associated fibroblasts (CAFs), via the powerful influence of specific microRNAs on gene expression—Cutting edge cancer research from veterinary science confirms a direct mechanistic link between the loss of tumor-suppressive nicro-RNAs (miR27a), the upregulation of CCNG1 (Cyclin G1), and fibroblast-to-CAF activation [165]—revealing the cellular *crosstalk* as intimidating hyperactivity of the **Cyclin G1/Cdk/cMyc Axis** (in bodily *hostage-taken TAFs*) which in-turn shape the tumor microenvironment.

The survival benefits of DeltaRex-G monotherapy achieved in Stage 4 (metastatic) cancers highlight the importance of *Pathotropic tumor-targeting* as an **enabling nanotechnology** for both Active Cancer Surveillance and Precision Gene Delivery. The proactive tumor-targeting platform was important enough medically (and morally) to rescue and re-establish the gene-based medicine: to restore the circular plasmid DNA rings (genetic blueprints); to resurrect the FDA-approved CMC, regain formal sponsorship, raise sufficient funds, and enable certified cGMP bioproduction under academic *not-for-profit* humanitarian banners [21], while attaining formal FDA approval for *The BLESSED Protocol: Expanded Access for DeltaRex-G for Advanced Pancreatic Cancer and Sarcoma* (ClinicalTrials.gov Identifier: NCT04091295) [166]. **In restoring DeltaRex-G from desuetude to the cancer clinic in 2019 (Survive & Thrive)**, we are reminded that we once penned a cautionary yet *forward-looking statement* concerning clinical utility more than a decade ago, when we reviewed the *'Timely' Development of Rexin-G: first targeted injectable gene vector,* and reported on its clinical anti-cancer activity [78]:

> *It bears mentioning that each and every one of the clinical benefits achieved at the terminal edge of end-stage cancer can be magnified exponentially when proactive tumor-targeted hunter/killers like DeltaRex-G are permitted, and ultimately mandated by good medical practice, to be administered earlier in the course of a malignant disease—for, after all, that is how Outlaw Cancer Cells grow within us—exponentially!*

Annus Mirabilis 2019: This contemporary saga of biopharmaceutical action and adventure was attended *socially* by the beatification of Father Joseph Aveni, a publicized case study wherein DeltaRex-G monotherapy enabled a veritable late-stage cancer remission [81], and *clinically* by the restoration of DeltaRex-G, as tumor-targeted gene therapy for metastatic cancer patients. Alas, it is with great sadness and respect that we mark the passing of John Paul Levy, a friend and colleague (1960–2019), who worked with Hall and Gordon in biotechnology, CMC, and cGMP to address important issues of retroviral vector safety, painstakingly discerning and eliminating plasmid homologies with innovative *synthetic design engineering*, thereby creating the advanced 5th generation FDA-approved tumor-targeted gene therapy vector series, which historically bears his name [77]—John Levy worked diligently to ensure the plasmid DNA sequences of DeltaRex-G were faithfully restored to approved FDA-specifications and that the clinical lots of DeltaRex-G (with updated cGMP) were certified for potency and as high-titers in approved vector testing facilities at UC Davis; thus, we acknowledge and honor John Paul Levy as an unsung Hero and respected member of the Aveni medical mission (A-Team) to restore DeltaRex-G in 2019.

Acknowledgements

Summing it all up: (i) with the reconstitution of the original blueprints (plasmid DNA sequences) for **DeltaRex-G** genetically verified, (ii) the clinical sponsorship of DeltaGex-G formally restored to Dr. Gordon, (iii) the re-establishment of CMC & scalable cGMP with FDA-approved vector production and certification, and (iv) the **Return of DeltaRex-G** cancer therapy to active clinical status [166], we hereby acknowledge and extend our personal appreciations to Dexter Gaston, Director of the North County Biotechnology Incubator, Vista California; Dr. Austin Mogen of Corning Life Sciences, for technical assistance with the "hyper-flask" technologies; William Swaney, Director of the Vector Production Core Facilities at Cincinnati Children's Hospital Medical Center; and the *Aveni Foundation Bioengineering Support Team* (**Vista "A-Team"**): including, John Levy, Jesus Hernandez, Rebecca Reed, Alison Reed, Nicholas Hall, and Heather Gordon. Finally, we salute Dr. Sant P. Chawla and the clinical staff at the Sarcoma Oncology Clinic of Southern California, where informed and empowered cancer patients have a brand-new legal and life-affirming Right-to-Try.

Author details

Frederick L. Hall[1] and Erlinda M. Gordon[1,2]*

1 Delta Next-Gene, LLC, Santa Monica, CA, USA

2 Aveni Foundation, Santa Monica, CA, USA

*Address all correspondence to: egordon@deltanextgen.com

IntechOpen

References

[1] Gordon EM, Hall FL. Nanotechnology blooms, at last (Review). Oncology Reports. 2005;13: 1003–1007. DOI: 10.3892/or.13.6.1003

[2] Gordon EM, Hall FL. A Primer on Pathotropic Medicine. In: One Hundred Years of the FDA and the Future of Global Health. Brooklands New Media Ltd; 2007. p. 80–83.

[3] Yahya WRW, Taha S. Interpreting Melville's typee: A Victorian age journey to understanding savage and civilized societies. Pertanika Journal of Social Science and Humanities. 2013;21: 201–212.

[4] Ma B, Wells A, Clark AM. The pan-therapeutic resistance of disseminated tumor cells: Role of phenotypic plasticity and the metastatic microenvironment. Seminars in Cancer Biology. 2020;60:138–147. DOI: 10.1016/j.semcancer.2019.07.021

[5] Carlson P, Dasgupta A, Grzelak CA, et al. Targeting the perivascular niche sensitizes disseminated tumour cells to chemotherapy. Nature Cell Biology. 2019;21:238–250. DOI: 10.1038/s41556-018-0267-0

[6] The Atlantic. The Disingenuousness of 'Right to Try' The New Law Has a Catchy Name, But it Will Only Make it More Difficult to Know if Medication is Effective or Safe [Internet]. 2018. Available from: https://www.theatlantic.com/health/archive/2018/06/right-to-try/561770 [Accessed: 2020-11-23]

[7] Carrieri D, Peccatori FA, Boniolo G. The ethical plausibility of the 'Right To Try' laws. Critical Reviews in Oncology/Hematology. 2018;122:64–71. DOI: 10.1016/j.critrevonc.2017.12.014

[8] Odom LF, Gordon EM. Acute monoblastic leukemia in infancy and early childhood: Successful treatment with an epipodophyllotoxin. Blood. 1984;64:875–882. DOI: 10.1182/blood.V64.4.875.875

[9] USC News. Hope Chest [Internet]. 1998. Available from: https://news.usc.edu/9843/Hope-Chest [Accessed 2020-11-23]

[10] USC News. USC Scientist Proposes a First — Gene Therapy In Utero [Internet]. 1998. Available from: https://news.usc.edu/9951/USC-Scientist-Proposes-a-First-Gene-Therapy-In-Utero [Accessed: 2020-11-21]

[11] Marsa L, McDougal D. The tangled life of William Anderson French: Sexual abuse charges cast a shadow on the "father of gene therapy" and bring new attention to questions about the research that made him famous. Los Angeles Magazine. 2005;50:116–121.

[12] Brown B, Ortiz C, Dubé K. Assessment of the Right-to-Try law: The pros and the cons. Journal of Nuclear Medicine. 2018;59:1492–1493. DOI: 10.2967/jnumed.118.216945

[13] Bateman-House A, Robertson CT. The federal Right to Try Act of 2017-a wrong turn for access to investigational drugs and the path forward. JAMA Internal Medicine. 2018;178:321–322. DOI: 10.1001/jamainternmed.2017.8167

[14] Fiori ME, Di Franco S, Villanova L, Bianca P, Stassi G, De Maria R. Cancer-associated fibroblasts as abettors of tumor progression at the crossroads of EMT and therapy resistance. Molecular Cancer. 2019;18:70. DOI: 10.1186/s12943-019-0994-2

[15] Waehler R, Russell SJ, Curiel DT. Engineering targeted viral vectors for gene therapy. Nature Reviews Genetic. 2007;8:573–587. DOI: 10.1038/nrg2141

[16] GEN - Genetic Engineering and Biotechnology News. The RAC Retires

after a Job Well Done [Internet]. 2019. Available from: https://www.genengne ws.com/insights/the-rac-retires-after-a-job-well-done/ [Accessed: 2020-11-23]

[17] Gordon EM, Chan MT, Geraldino N, Lopez FF, Cornelio GH, Lorenzo CC, Levy JP, Reed RA, Liu L, Hall FL. Le morte du tumour: Histological features of tumor destruction in chemo-resistant cancers following intravenous infusions of pathotropic nanoparticles bearing therapeutic genes. International Journal of Oncology. 2007;30:1297–1307. DOI: 10.3892/ijo.30.6.1297

[18] Gordon EM, Hall FL. Rexin-G, a targeted genetic medicine for cancer. Expert Opinion on Biological Therapy. 2010;10:819–832. DOI: 10.1517/ 14712598.2010.481666

[19] Gordon EM, Hall FL. Critical stages in the development of the first targeted, injectable molecular-genetic medicine for cancer. In: Kang C, editor. Gene Therapy Applications. InTech; 2011. p. 461–492. DOI: 10.5772/21120.

[20] Gordon EM, Ravicz JR, Liu S, Chawla SP, Hall FL. Cell cycle checkpoint control: The cyclin G1/ Mdm2/p53 axis emerges as a strategic target for broad-spectrum cancer gene therapy - A review of molecular mechanisms for oncologists. Molecular and Clinical Oncology. 2018;9:115–134. DOI: 10.3892/mco.2018.1657

[21] Cancer Therapy Advisor. The Revival of a Forgotten Cancer Gene Therapy with Off-the-Shelf Potential [Internet]. 2019. Available from: https:// www.cancertherapyadvisor.com/home/ cancer-topics/general-oncology/forgotte n-cancer-gene-therapy-revival-with-off-shelf-potential [Accessed: 2020-11-01]

[22] Lui SY, Chawla SP, Bruckner H, Morse MA, Federman N, Ignacio JG, San Juan F, Manalo RA, Hall FL, Gordon EM. Reporting long term survival following precision tumor-targeted gene delivery to advanced chemotherapy-resistant malignancies: An academic milestone. Cell Press. 2019; 27:133.

[23] Hall FL, Gordon EM, Wu L, Zhu NL, Skotzko MJ, Starnes VA, Anderson WF. Targeting retroviral vectors to vascular lesions by genetic engineering of the MoMLV gp70 envelope protein. Human Gene Therapy. 1997;8:2183–2192. DOI: 10.1089/hum.1997.8.18-2183

[24] Hall FL, Liu L, Zhu NL, Stapfer M, Anderson WF, Beart RW, Gordon EM. Molecular engineering of matrix-targeted retroviral vectors incorporating a surveillance function inherent in von Willebrand factor. Human Gene Therapy. 2000;11:983–993. DOI: 10.1089/10430340050015293

[25] Zhu NL, Gordon EM, Terramani T, Anderson WF, Hall FL. Collagen-targeted retroviral vectors displaying domain D2 of von Willebrand factor (vWF-D2) enhance gene transfer to human tissue explants. International Journal of Pediatric Hematology-Oncology 2001;7:325–335.

[26] Gordon EM, Zhu NL, Forney Prescott M, Zhen HC, Anderson WF, Hall FL. Lesion-Targeted Injectable Vectors for Vascular Restenosis. Human Gene Therapy. 2001;12:1277–1287. DOI: 10.1089/104303401750270931

[27] Gomis RR, Gawrzak S. Tumor cell dormancy. Molecular Oncology. 2017; 11:62–78. DOI: 10.1016/j. molonc.2016.09.009

[28] Endo H, Inoue M. Dormancy in cancer. Cancer Science. 2019;110:474–480. DOI: 10.1111/cas.13917

[29] Gimbrone MA Jr, Leapman SB, Cotran RS, Folkman J. Tumor dormancy in vivo by prevention of neovascularization. The Journal of

Experimental Medicine. 1972;136:261–276. DOI: 10.1084/jem.136.2.261

[30] Osisami M, Keller ET. Mechanisms of metastatic tumor dormancy. Journal of Clinical Medicine. 2013;2:136–150. DOI: 10.3390/jcm2030136

[31] Fernandes C, Suares D, Yergeri MC. Tumor microenvironment targeted nanotherapy. Frontiers in Pharmacology. 2018;9:1230. DOI: 10.3389/fphar.2018.01230

[32] Nissen NI, Karsdal M, Willumsen N. Collagens and cancer associated fibroblasts in the reactive stroma and its relation to cancer biology. Journal of Experimental & Clinical Cancer Research. 2019;38:115. DOI: 10.1186/s13046-019-1110-6

[33] Nerenberg PS, Salsas-Escat R, Stultz CM. Collagen – a necessary accomplice in the metastatic process. Cancer Genomics & Proteomics. 2007;4:319–328.

[34] Werner-Klein M, Klein CA. Therapy resistance beyond cellular dormancy. Nature Cell Biology. 2019;21:117–119. DOI: 10.1038/s41556-019-0276-7

[35] Tuan TL, Cheung DT, Wu LT, Yee A, Gabriel S, Han B, Morton L, Nimni ME, Hall FL. Engineering, expression and renaturation of targeted TGF-beta fusion proteins. Connective Tissue Research. 1996;34:1–9. DOI: 10.3109/03008209609028888

[36] Andrades JA, Nimni ME, Han B, Ertl DC, Hall FL, Becerra J. Type I collagen combined with a recombinant TGF-beta serves as a scaffold for mesenchymal stem cells. The International Journal of Developmental Biology. 1996;Suppl 1:107S–108S.

[37] Andrades JA, Han B, Becerra J, Sorgente N, Hall FL, Nimni ME. A recombinant human TGF-beta1 fusion protein with collagen-binding domain promotes migration, growth, and differentiation of bone marrow mesenchymal cells. Experimental Cell Research. 1999;250:485–498. DOI: 10.1006/excr.1999.4528

[38] Han B, Perelman N, Tang B, Hall F, Shors EC, Nimni ME. Collagen-targeted BMP3 fusion proteins arrayed on collagen matrices or porous ceramics impregnated with Type I collagen enhance osteogenesis in a rat cranial defect model. Journal of Orthopaedic Research: Official Publication of the Orthopaedic Research Society. 2002;20:747–755. DOI: 10.1016/S0736-0266(01)00157-7

[39] Gordon EM, Skotzko M, Kundu RK, Han B, Andrades J, Nimni M, Anderson WF, Hall FL. Capture and expansion of bone marrow-derived mesenchymal progenitor cells with a transforming growth factor-beta1-von Willebrand's factor fusion protein for retrovirus-mediated delivery of coagulation factor IX. Human Gene Therapy. 1997;8:1385–1394. DOI: 10.1089/hum.1997.8.11-1385

[40] Hall FL, Han B, Kundu RK, Yee A, Nimni ME, Gordon EM. Phenotypic differentiation of TGF-beta1-responsive pluripotent premesenchymal prehematopoietic progenitor (P4 stem) cells from murine bone marrow. Journal of Hematotherapy & Stem Cell Research. 2001;10:261–271. DOI: 10.1089/15258160151134962

[41] Reiser J, Zhang XY, Hemenway CS, Mondal D, Pradhan L, La Russa VF. Potential of mesenchymal stem cells in gene therapy approaches for inherited and acquired diseases. Expert Opinion on Biological Therapy. 2005;5:1571–1584. DOI: 10.1517/14712598.5.12.1571

[42] Hall FL, Kaiser A, Liu L, Chen ZH, Hu J, Nimni ME, Beart RW Jr, Gordon EM. Design, expression, and renaturation of a lesion-targeted

recombinant epidermal growth factor-von Willebrand factor fusion protein: efficacy in an animal model of experimental colitis. International Journal of Molecular Medicine. 2000;6: 635–643. DOI: 10.3892/ijmm.6.6.635

[43] Pyagay P, Heroult M, Wang Q, Lehnert W, Belden J, Liaw L, Friesel RE, Lindner V. Collagen Triple Helix Repeat Containing 1, a Novel Secreted Protein in Injured and Diseased Arteries, Inhibits Collagen Expression and Promotes Cell Migration. Circulation Research. 2005;96:261–268. DOI: 10.1161/01.RES.0000154262.07264.12

[44] Zhang R, Cao Y, Bai L, Zhu C, Li R, Liu Y, Wu K, Liu F, Wu J. The collagen triple helix repeat containing 1 facilitates hepatitis B virus-associated hepatocellular carcinoma progression by regulating multiple cellular factors and signal cascades. Molecular Carcinogenesis. 2015;54:1554–1566. DOI: 10.1002/mc.22229

[45] Tang L, Dai DL, Su M, Martinka M, Li G, Zhou Y. Aberrant expression of collagen triple helix repeat containing 1 in human solid cancers. Clinical Cancer Research. 2006;12:3716–3722. DOI: 10.1158/1078-0432.CCR-06-0030

[46] Park EH, Kim S, Jo JY, Kim SJ, Hwang Y, Kim JM, Song SY, Lee DK, Koh SS. Collagen triple helix repeat containing-1 promotes pancreatic cancer progression by regulating migration and adhesion of tumor cells. Carcinogenesis. 2013;34:694–702. DOI: 10.1093/carcin/bgs378

[47] Jiang N, Cui Y, Liu J, Zhu X, Wu H, Yang Z, Ke Z. Multidimensional Roles of Collagen Triple Helix Repeat Containing 1 (CTHRC1) in Malignant Cancers. Journal of Cancer. 2016;7:2213–2220. DOI: 10.7150/jca.16539

[48] He W, Zhang H, Wang Y, Zhou Y, Luo Y, Cui Y, Jiang N, Jiang W, Wang H, Xu D, Li S, Wang Z, Chen Y,

Sun Y, Zhang Y, Tseng HR, Zou X, Wang L, Ke Z. CTHRC1 induces non-small cell lung cancer (NSCLC) invasion through upregulating MMP-7/MMP-9. BMC Cancer. 2018;18:400. DOI: 10.1186/s12885-018-4317-6

[49] Fang M, Yuan J, Peng C, Li Y. Collagen as a double-edged sword in tumor progression. Tumour Biology: The Journal of the International Society for Oncodevelopmental Biology and Medicine. 2014;35:2871–2882. DOI: 10.1007/s13277-013-1511-7

[50] Manka SW, Bihan D, Farndale RW. Structural studies of the MMP-3 interaction with triple-helical collagen introduce new roles for the enzyme in tissue remodelling. Scientific Reports. 2019;9:18785. DOI: 10.1038/s41598-019-55266-9

[51] Eriksson J, Le Joncour V, Nummela P, Jahkola T, Virolainen S, Laakkonen P, Saksela O, Hölttä E. Gene expression analyses of primary melanomas reveal CTHRC1 as an important player in melanoma progression. Oncotarget. 2016;7: 15065–15092. DOI: 10.18632/oncotarget.7604

[52] Xu J, Rodriguez D, Petitclerc E, Kim JJ, Hangai M, Moon YS, Davis GE, Brooks PC. Proteolytic exposure of a cryptic site within collagen type IV is required for angiogenesis and tumor growth in vivo. Journal of Cell Biology. 2001;154:1069–1080. DOI: 10.1083/jcb.200103111

[53] Turkar S, Ramaswamy A, Ostwal V. A step ahead on CTHRC1, and not just reinventing the wheel! Chinese Clinical Oncology. 2019;8:S17. DOI: 10.21037/cco.2019.02.05

[54] Orgel JP, Antipova O, Sagi I, Bitler A, Qiu D, Wang R, Xu Y, San Antonio JD. Collagen fibril surface displays a constellation of sites capable of promoting fibril assembly, stability,

and hemostasis. Connective Tissue Research. 2011;52:18–24. DOI: 10.3109/03008207.2010.511354

[55] Hoop CL, Zhu J, Nunes AM, Case DA, Baum J. Revealing accessibility of cryptic protein binding sites within the functional collagen fibril. Biomolecules. 2017;7:4. DOI: 10.3390/biom7040076.

[56] Goldbloom-Helzner L, Hao D, Wang A. Developing Regenerative Treatments for Developmental Defects, Injuries, and Diseases Using Extracellular Matrix Collagen-Targeting Peptides. International Journal of Molecular Sciences. 2019;20:17. DOI: 10.3390/ijms20174072.

[57] Provenzano PP, Eliceiri KW, Campbell JM, Inman DR, White JG, Keely PJ. Collagen reorganization at the tumor-stromal interface facilitates local invasion. BMC Medicine. 2006;4:38. DOI: 10.1186/1741-7015-4-38

[58] Karagiannis GS, Petraki C, Prassas I, Saraon P, Musrap N, Dimitromanolakis A, Diamandis EP. Proteomic signatures of the desmoplastic invasion front reveal collagen type XII as a marker of myofibroblastic differentiation during colorectal cancer metastasis. Oncotarget. 2012;3:267–285. DOI: 10.18632/oncotarget.451

[59] Hall FL, Levy JP, Reed RA, Wasinee NP, Chua VS, Chawla SP, Gordon EM. Pathotropic targeting advances clinical oncology: Tumor-targeted localization of therapeutic gene delivery. Oncology Reports. 2010;24:829–833. DOI: 10.3892/or_00000926

[60] Tjomsland V, Niklasson L, Sandström P, Borch K, Druid H, Bratthäll C, Messmer D, Larsson M, Spångeus A. The desmoplastic stroma plays an essential role in the accumulation and modulation of infiltrated immune cells in pancreatic adenocarcinoma. Clinical & Developmental Immunology. 2011;2011:212810. DOI: 10.1155/2011/212810

[61] Watt J, Kocher HM. The desmoplastic stroma of pancreatic cancer is a barrier to immune cell infiltration. Oncoimmunology. 2013;2:12. DOI: 10.4161/onci.26788.

[62] Guo FF, Cui JW. The role of tumor-infiltrating B cells in tumor immunity. Journal of Oncology. 2019;2019:2592419. DOI: 10.1155/2019/2592419

[63] Muppa P, Parrilha Terra SBS, Sharma A, Mansfield AS, Aubry MC, Bhinge K, Asiedu MK, de Andrade M, Janaki N, Murphy SJ, Nasir A, Van Keulen V, Vasmatzis G, Wigle DA, Yang P, Yi ES, Peikert T, Kosari F. Immune cell infiltration may be a key determinant of long-term survival in small cell lung cancer. Journal of Thoracic Oncology. 2019;14:1286–1295. DOI: 10.1016/j.jtho.2019.03.028

[64] Sultan M, Coyle KM, Vidovic D, Thomas ML, Gujar S, Marcato P. Hide-and-seek: The interplay between cancer stem cells and the immune system. Carcinogenesis. 2017;38:107–118. DOI: 10.1186/s13027-016-0085-6

[65] Abdollahi A, Folkman J. Evading tumor evasion: current concepts and perspectives of anti-angiogenic cancer therapy. Drug Resistance Updates: Reviews and Commentaries in Antimicrobial and Anticancer Chemotherapy. 2010;13:16–28. DOI: 10.1016/j.drup.2009.12.001

[66] Jászai J, Schmidt MHH. Trends and challenges in tumor anti-angiogenic therapies. Cells. 2019;8:1102. DOI: 10.3390/cells8091102.

[67] Yuan S, Norgard RJ, Stanger BZ. Cellular Plasticity in Cancer. Cancer Discovery. 2019;9:837–851. DOI: 10.1158/2159-8290.CD-19-0015

[68] Maeda H, Khatami M. Analyses of repeated failures in cancer therapy for solid tumors: poor tumor-selective drug delivery, low therapeutic efficacy and unsustainable costs. Clinical and Translational Medicine. 2018;7:e11. DOI: 10.1186/s40169-018-0185-6

[69] Roma-Rodrigues C, Mendes R, Baptista PV, Fernandes AR. Targeting tumor microenvironment for cancer therapy. International Journal of Molecular Sciences. 2019;20:4. DOI: 10.3390/ijms20040840.

[70] Tsai MJ, Chang WA, Huang MS, Kuo PL. Tumor microenvironment: a new treatment target for cancer. ISRN Biochemistry. 2014;2014:351959. DOI: 10.1155/2014/351959

[71] Kozlova N, Grossman JE, Iwanicki MP, Muranen T. The interplay of the extracellular matrix and stromal cells as a drug target in stroma-rich cancers. Trends in Pharmacological Sciences. 2020;41:183–198. DOI: 10.1016/j.tips.2020.01.001

[72] Nam J, Son S, Park KS, Zou W, Shea LD, Moon JJ. Cancer nanomedicine for combination cancer immunotherapy. Nature Reviews Materials. 2019;4:398–414. DOI: 10.1038/s41578-019-0108-1

[73] Gordon EM, Liu PX, Chen ZH, Liu L, Whitley MD, Gee C, Groshen S, Hinton DR, Beart RW, Hall FL. Inhibition of metastatic tumor growth in nude mice by portal vein infusions of matrix-targeted retroviral vectors bearing a cytocidal cyclin G1 construct. Cancer Research. 2000;60: 3343–3347.

[74] Gordon EM, Chen ZH, Liu L, Whitley M, Liu L, Wei D, Groshen S, Hinton DR, Anderson WF, Beart RW Jr, Hall FL. Systemic administration of a matrix-targeted retroviral vector is efficacious for cancer gene therapy in mice. Human Gene Therapy. 2001;12:

193–204. DOI: 10.1089/104303401750061258

[75] Lenz HJ, Anderson WF, Hall FL, Gordon EM. Clinical protocol. Tumor site specific phase I evaluation of safety and efficacy of hepatic arterial infusion of a matrix-targeted retroviral vector bearing a dominant negative cyclin G1 construct as intervention for colorectal carcinoma metastatic to liver. Human Gene Therapy. 2002;13:1515–1537. DOI: 10.1089/10430340260185148

[76] Gordon EM, Lopez FF, Cornelio GH, Lorenzo CC 3rd, Levy JP, Reed RA, Liu L, Bruckner HW, Hall FL. Pathotropic nanoparticles for cancer gene therapy Rexin-G IV: three-year clinical experience. International Journal of Oncology. 2006;29:1053–1064.

[77] Gordon EM, Levy JP, Reed RA, Petchpud WN, Liu L, Wendler CB, Hall FL. Targeting metastatic cancer from the inside: a new generation of targeted gene delivery vectors enables personalized cancer vaccination in situ. International Journal of Oncology. 2008; 33:665–675.

[78] Gordon EM, Hall FL. The 'timely' development of Rexin-G: first targeted injectable gene vector (review). International Journal of Oncology. 2009; 35:229–238.

[79] Chawla SP, Chua VS, Fernandez L, Quon D, Saralou A, Blackwelder WC, Hall FL, Gordon EM. Phase I/II and Phase II Studies of Targeted Gene Delivery In Vivo: Intravenous Rexin-G for Chemotherapy-resistant Sarcoma and Osteosarcoma. Molecular Therapy. 2009;17:1651–1657. DOI: 10.1038/mt.2009.126

[80] Chawla SP, Chua VS, Fernandez L, Quon D, Blackwelder WC, Gordon EM, Hall FL. Advanced Phase I/II Studies of Targeted Gene Delivery In Vivo: Intravenous Rexin-G for Gemcitabine-resistant Metastatic Pancreatic Cancer.

Molecular Therapy. 2010;18:435–441. DOI: 10.1038/mt.2009.228

[81] Gordon EM, Hall FL. Noteworthy clinical case studies in cancer gene therapy: Tumor-targeted Rexin-G advances as an efficacious anti-cancer agent. International Journal of Oncology. 2010;36:1341–1353. DOI: 10.3892/ijo_00000619

[82] Chawla SP, Bruckner H, Morse MA, Assudani N, Hall FL, Gordon EM. A Phase I-II Study Using Rexin-G Tumor-Targeted Retrovector Encoding a Dominant-Negative Cyclin G1 Inhibitor for Advanced Pancreatic Cancer. Molecular Therapy Oncolytics. 2019;12: 56–67. DOI: 10.1016/j.omto.2018.12.005

[83] Al-Shihabi A, Chawla SP, Hall FL, Gordon EM. Exploiting Oncogenic Drivers along the CCNG1 Pathway for Cancer Therapy and Gene Therapy. Molecular Therapy Oncolytics. 2018;11: 122–126. DOI: 10.1016/j.omto.2018.11.002

[84] Reimer CL, Borras AM, Kurdistani SK, Garreau JR, Chung M, Aaronson SA, Lee SW. Altered regulation of cyclin G in human breast cancer and its specific localization at replication foci in response to DNA damage in p53+/+ cells. The Journal of Biological Chemistry. 1999;274:11022–11029. DOI: 10.1074/jbc.274.16.11022

[85] Perez R, Wu N, Klipfel AA, Beart Jr. RW, Costello CW, Costello C. A better cell cycle target for gene therapy of colorectal cancer: Cyclin G. Journal of Gastrointestinal Surgery. 2003;7:884–889. DOI: 10.1007/s11605-003-0034-8

[86] Alsinet C, Villanueva A, Llovet JM. Cell population genetics and deep sequencing: a novel approach for drivers discovery in hepatocellular carcinoma. Journal of Hepatology. 2012;56:1198–1200. DOI: 10.1016/j.jhep.2011.11.014

[87] Russell P, Hennessy BT, Li J, Carey MS, Bast RC, Freeman T, Venkitaraman AR. Cyclin G1 regulates the outcome of taxane-induced mitotic checkpoint arrest. Oncogene. 2012;31: 2450–2460. DOI: 10.1038/onc.2011.431

[88] Shang Y, Feng B, Zhou L, Ren G, Zhang Z, Fan X, Sun Y, Luo G, Liang J, Wu K, Nie Y, Fan D. The miR27b-CCNG1-P53-miR-508-5p axis regulates multidrug resistance of gastric cancer. Oncotarget. 2016;7:538–549. DOI: 10.18632/oncotarget.6374

[89] Fornari F, Gramantieri L, Giovannini C, Veronese A, Ferracin M, Sabbioni S, Calin GA, Grazi GL, Croce CM, Tavolari S, Chieco P, Negrini M, Bolondi L. MiR-122/cyclin G1 interaction modulates p53 activity and affects doxorubicin sensitivity of human hepatocarcinoma cells. Cancer Research. 2009;69:5761–5767. DOI: 10.1158/0008-5472.CAN-08-4797

[90] Ma L, Liu J, Shen J, Liu L, Wu J, Li W, Luo J, Chen Q, Qian C. Expression of miR-122 mediated by adenoviral vector induces apoptosis and cell cycle arrest of cancer cells. Cancer Biology & Therapy. 2010;9:554–561. DOI: 10.4161/cbt.9.7.11267

[91] Qin H, Sha J, Jiang C, Gao X, Qu L, Yan H, Xu T, Jiang Q, Gao H. miR-122 inhibits metastasis and epithelial–mesenchymal transition of non-small-cell lung cancer cells. OncoTargets and Therapy. 2015;8:3175–3184. DOI: 10.2147/OTT.S91696

[92] Pan C, Wang X, Shi K, Zheng Y, Li J, Chen Y, Jin L, Pan Z. MiR-122 Reverses the Doxorubicin-Resistance in Hepatocellular Carcinoma Cells through Regulating the Tumor Metabolism. PLoS One. 2016;11:e0152090. DOI: 10.1371/journal.pone.0152090.

[93] Xu Y, Zhang Q, Miao C, Dongol S, Li Y, Jin C, Dong R, Li Y, Yang X, Kong B. CCNG1 (Cyclin G1) regulation by mutant-P53 via induction of Notch3 expression promotes high-grade serous

ovarian cancer (HGSOC) tumorigenesis and progression. Cancer Medicine. 2018;8:351–362. DOI: 10.1002/cam4.1812

[94] Luan Y, Han T, Liu R, Yang X, Li Q. Cyclin G1 mediates the poor prognosis of breast cancer through expanding the cancer stem cells. International Journal of Clinical and Experimental Medicine. 2019;12:5475–5486.

[95] Boix L, López-Oliva JM, Rhodes AC, Bruix J. Restoring miR122 in human stem-like hepatocarcinoma cells, prompts tumor dormancy through Smad-independent TGF-β pathway. Oncotarget. 2016;7:71309–71329. DOI: 10.18632/oncotarget.11885

[96] Wu L, Liu L, Yee A, Carbonarohall D, Tolo VT, Hall FL. Molecular cloning of the human CYCG1 gene encoding a G-type cyclin: Overexpression in human osteosarcoma cells. Oncology Reports. 1994;1:705–711. DOI: 10.3892/or.1.4.705

[97] Horne MC, Goolsby GL, Donaldson KL, Tran D, Neubauer M, Wahl AF. Cyclin G1 and cyclin G2 comprise a new family of cyclins with contrasting tissue-specific and cell cycle-regulated expression. Journal of Biological Chemistry. 1996;271:6050–6061. DOI: 10.1074/jbc.271.11.6050

[98] Chen DS, Zhu N-L, Hung G, Skotzko MJ, Hinton DR, Tolo V, Hall FL, Anderson WF, Gordon EM. Retroviral vector-mediated transfer of an antisense cyclin G1 construct inhibits osteosarcoma tumor growth in nude mice. Human Gene Therapy. 2008;8:1667–1674. DOI: 10.1089/hum.1997.8.14-1667

[99] Xu F, Wang Y, Hall FL. Molecular cloning and characterization of FX3, a novel zinc-finger protein. Oncology Reports. 2000;7:995–1001.

[100] Cuadrado A, Lafarga V, Cheung PC, Dolado I, Llanos S,

Cohen P, Nebreda AR. A new p38 MAP kinase-regulated transcriptional coactivator that stimulates p53-dependent apoptosis. The EMBO Journal. 2007;26:2115–2126. DOI: 10.1038/sj.emboj.7601657

[101] Vousden KH, Prives C. Blinded by the Light: The Growing Complexity of p53. Cell. 2009;137:413–431. DOI: 10.1016/j.cell.2009.04.037

[102] Lafarga V, Cuadrado A, Nebreda AR. p18Hamlet mediates different p53-dependent responses to DNA damage inducing agents. Cell Cycle. 2007;6:2319–2322. DOI: 10.4161/cc.6.19.4741

[103] Cuadrado A, Corrado N, Perdiguero E, Lafarga V, Muñoz-Canoves P, Nebreda AR. Essential role of p18Hamlet/SRCAP-mediated histone H2A.Z chromatin incorporation in muscle differentiation. The EMBO Journal. 2010;29:2014–2025. DOI: 10.1038/emboj.2010.85

[104] Weinstein IB, Joe AK. Mechanisms of disease: Oncogene addiction–a rationale for molecular targeting in cancer therapy. Nature Clinical Practice. Oncology. 2006;3:448–457. DOI: 10.1038/ncponc0558

[105] Torti D, Trusolino L. Oncogene addiction as a foundational rationale for targeted anti-cancer therapy: Promises and perils. EMBO Molecular Medicine. 2011;3:623–636. DOI: 10.1002/emmm.201100176

[106] Gramantieri L, Ferracin M, Fornari F, Veronese A, Sabbioni S, Liu CG, Calin GA, Giovannini C, Ferrazzi E, Grazi GL, Croce CM, Bolondi L, Negrini M. Cyclin G1 is a target of miR-122a, a microRNA frequently down-regulated in human hepatocellular carcinoma. Cancer Research. 2007;67:6092–6099. DOI: 10.1158/0008-5472. CAN-06-4607

[107] Yan J, Jiang JY, Meng XN, Xiu YL, Zong ZH. MiR-23b targets cyclin G1 and suppresses ovarian cancer tumorigenesis and progression. Journal of Experimental & Clinical Cancer Research. 2016;35:31. DOI: 10.1186/s13046-016-0307-1

[108] Huang CS, Chu J, Zhu XX, Li JH, Huang XT, Cai JP, Zhao W, Yin XY. The C/EBPβ-LINC01133 axis promotes cell proliferation in pancreatic ductal adenocarcinoma through upregulation of CCNG1. Cancer Letters. 2018;421: 63–72. DOI: 10.1016/j.canlet. 2018.02.020

[109] Hall FL, Vulliet PR. Proline-directed protein phosphorylation and cell cycle regulation. Current Opinion in Cell Biology. 1991;3:176–184. DOI: 10.1016/0955-0674(91)90136-m

[110] Hall FL, Mitchell JP, Vulliet PR. Phosphorylation of synapsin I at a novel site by proline-directed protein kinase. The Journal of Biological Chemistry. 1990;265:6944–6948.

[111] Williams R, Sanghera J, Wu F, Carbonaro-Hall D, Campbell DL, Warburton D, Pelech S, Hall F. Identification of a human epidermal growth factor receptor-associated protein kinase as a new member of the mitogen-activated protein kinase/extracellular signal-regulated protein kinase family. The Journal of Biological Chemistry. 1993;268:18213–18217.

[112] Sanghera JS, Hall FL, Warburton D, Campbell D, Pelech SL. Identification of epidermal growth factor Thr-669 phosphorylation site peptide kinases as distinct MAP kinases and p34cdc2. Biochimica et Biophysica Acta (BBA) - Molecular Cell Research. 1992;1135:335–342. DOI: 10.1016/0167-4889(92) 90240-C

[113] Gordon EM, Venkatesan N, Salazar R, Tang H, Schmeidler-Sapiro K, Buckley S, Warburton D, Hall FL. Factor XII-induced mitogenesis is mediated via a distinct signal transduction pathway that activates a mitogen-activated protein kinase. Proceedings of the National Academy of Sciences of the United States of America. 1996;93:2174–2179.

[114] Peeper DS, Parker LL, Ewen ME, Toebes M, Hall FL, Xu M, Zantema A, van der Eb AJ, Piwnica-Worms H. A- and B-type cyclins differentially modulate substrate specificity of cyclin-cdk complexes. The EMBO Journal. 1993;12:1947–1954.

[115] Elledge SJ, Richman R, Hall FL, Williams RT, Lodgson N, Harper JW. CDK2 encodes a 33-kDa cyclin A-associated protein kinase and is expressed before CDC2 in the cell cycle. Proceedings of the National Academy of Sciences of the United States of America. 1992;89:2907–2911. DOI: 10.1073/pnas.89.7.2907

[116] Hall FL, Williams RT, Wu L, Wu F, Carbonaro-Hall DA, Harper JW, Warburton D. Two potentially oncogenic cyclins, cyclin A and cyclin D1, share common properties of subunit configuration, tyrosine phosphorylation and physical association with the Rb protein. Oncogene. 1993;8:1377–1384.

[117] Hall F, Morita M, Best JB. Neoplastic transformation in the planarian: I. Cocarcinogenesis and histopathology. Journal of Experimental Zoology. 1986;240:211–227. DOI: 10.1002/jez.1402400209

[118] Hall F, Morita M, Best JB. Neoplastic transformation in the planarian: II. Ultrastructure of malignant reticuloma. Journal of Experimental Zoology. 1986;240:229–244. DOI: 10.1002/jez.1402400210

[119] Bayer FE, Zimmermann M, Fischer P, Gromoll C, Preiss A, Nagel AC. p53 and cyclin G cooperate in

mediating genome stability in somatic cells of Drosophila. Scientific Reports. 2017;7:17890. DOI: 10.1038/s41598-017-17973-z

[120] Hartl M. The quest for targets executing MYC-dependent cell transformation. Frontiers in Oncology. 2016;6:132. DOI: 10.3389/fonc.2016.00132.

[121] Yoshida GJ. Emerging roles of Myc in stem cell biology and novel tumor therapies. Journal of Experimental & Clinical Cancer Research. 2018;37:173. DOI: 10.1186/s13046-018-0835-y

[122] García-Gutiérrez L, Delgado MD, León J. MYC oncogene contributions to release of cell cycle brakes. Genes. 2019; 10:3. DOI: 10.3390/genes10030244.

[123] Carabet LA, Rennie PS, Cherkasov A. Therapeutic inhibition of Myc in cancer. Structural bases and computer-aided drug discovery approaches. International Journal of Molecular Sciences. 2018;20:120. DOI: 10.3390/ijms20010120.

[124] Allen-Petersen BL, Sears RC. Mission possible: Advances in MYC therapeutic targeting in cancer. BioDrugs. 2019;33:539-553. DOI: 10.1007/s40259-019-00370-5

[125] Seo HR, Kim J, Bae S, Soh JW, Lee YS. Cdk5-mediated Phosphorylation of c-Myc on Ser-62 Is Essential in Transcriptional Activation of Cyclin B1 by Cyclin G1. Journal of Biological Chemistry. 2008;283:15601-15610. DOI: 10.1074/jbc.M800987200

[126] Zhang X, Wang J, Jia Y, Liu T, Wang M, Lv W, Zhang R, Shi J, Liu L. CDK5 neutralizes the tumor suppressing effect of BIN1 via mediating phosphorylation of c-MYC at Ser-62 site in NSCLC. Cancer Cell International. 2019;19:226. DOI: 10.1186/s12935-019-0952-5

[127] O'Neill CP, Dwyer RM. Nanoparticle-based delivery of tumor suppressor microRNA for cancer therapy. Cells. 2020;9:2. DOI: 10.3390/cells9020521.

[128] Horiuchi D, Anderton B, Goga A. Taking on challenging targets: Making MYC druggable. American Society of Clinical Oncology Educational Book. 2014;e497–e502. DOI: 10.14694/EdBook_AM.2014.34.e497

[129] DeGregori J. Evolved tumor suppression: why are we so good at not getting cancer? Cancer Research. 2011; 71:3739–3744. DOI: 10.1158/0008-5472.CAN-11-0342

[130] Abegglen LM, Caulin AF, Chan A, Lee K, Robinson R, Campbell MS, Kiso WK, Schmitt DL, Waddell PJ, Bhaskara S, Jensen ST, Maley CC, Schiffman JD. Potential mechanisms for cancer resistance in elephants and comparative cellular response to DNA damage in humans. Journal of the American Medical Association. 2015; 314:1850–1860. DOI: 10.1001/jama.2015.13134

[131] Sulak M, Fong L, Mika K, Chigurupati S, Yon L, Mongan NP, Emes RD, Lynch VJ. TP53 copy number expansion is associated with the evolution of increased body size and an enhanced DNA damage response in elephants. Elife. 2016;5:e11994. DOI: 10.7554/eLife.11994.

[132] Stein Y, Rotter V, Aloni-Grinstein R. Gain-of-function mutant p53: All the roads lead to tumorigenesis. International Journal of Molecular Sciences. 2019;20: 24. DOI: 10.3390/ijms20246197.

[133] Li H, Okamoto K, Peart MJ, Prives C. Lysine-Independent Turnover of Cyclin G1 Can Be Stabilized by B'α Subunits of Protein Phosphatase 2A. Molecular and Cellular Biology. 2009; 29:919–928. DOI: 10.1128/MCB.00907-08

[134] Quandt E, Ribeiro MPC, Clotet J. Atypical cyclins: the extended family portrait. Cellular and Molecular Life Sciences. 2020;77:231–242. DOI: 10.1007/s00018-019-03262-7

[135] Canaud G, Brooks CR, Kishi S, Taguchi K, Nishimura K, Magassa S, Scott A, Hsiao LL, Ichimura T, Terzi F, Yang L, Bonventre JV. Cyclin G1 and TASCC regulate kidney epithelial cell G2-M arrest and fibrotic maladaptive repair. Science Translational Medicine. 2019;11:476. DOI: 10.1126/scitranslmed. aav4754.

[136] Hydbring P, Malumbres M, Sicinski P. Non-canonical functions of cell cycle cyclins and cyclin-dependent kinases. Nature Reviews Molecular Cell Biology. 2016;17:280–292. DOI: 10.1038/ nrm.2016.27

[137] Garnier L, Gkountidi A-O, Hugues S. Tumor-associated lymphatic vessel features and immunomodulatory functions. Frontiers in Immunology. 2019;10:720. DOI: 10.3389/ fimmu.2019.00720.

[138] Chawla SP, Chawla NS, Blackwelder WC, Hall FL, Gordon EM, Quon D, Chua-Alcala VS. An Advanced Phase 1/2 Study using an XC-Targeted Gene Therapy Vector for Chemotherapy Resistant Sarcoma. Sarcoma Research International. 2016;3:1–7.

[139] Kim S, Federman N, Gordon EM, Hall FL, Chawla SP. Rexin-G®, a tumor-targeted retrovector for malignant peripheral nerve sheath tumor: A case report. Molecular and Clinical Oncology. 2017;6:861–865. DOI: 10.3892/mco.2017.1231

[140] Juan FS, Manalo R, Nategh ES, Tamhane J, Kantamneni L, Chawla S, Hall F, Gordon E. The Genevieve protocol: Phase I/II evaluation of a dual targeted approach to cancer gene therapy/immunotherapy. Clinics in Oncology. 2018;3:1–7.

[141] Chawla SP, Bruckner H, Morse MA, Assudani N, Hall FL, Gordon EM. (repeated) A Phase I-II Study Using Rexin-G Tumor-Targeted Retrovector Encoding a Dominant-Negative Cyclin G1 Inhibitor for Advanced Pancreatic Cancer. Molecular Therapy Oncolytics. 2019;12:56–67. DOI: 10.1016/j.omto.2018.12.005

[142] Dy PSG, Hall FL, Chawla SP, Gordon EM. Immune cell trafficking in the tumor microenvironment of human cyclin G1 (CCNG1) inhibitor-treated tumors. British Journal of Cancer Research. 2018;1:202–207. DOI: 10.31488/bjcr.117.

[143] Kim S, Signorovitch JE, Yang H, Patterson-Lomba O, Xiang CQ, Ung B, Parisi M, Marshall JL. Comparative Effectiveness of nab-Paclitaxel Plus Gemcitabine vs FOLFIRINOX in Metastatic Pancreatic Cancer: A Retrospective Nationwide Chart Review in the United States. Advances in Therapy. 2018;35:1564–1577. DOI: 10.1007/s12325-018-0784-z

[144] Bewick V, Cheek L, Ball J. Statistics review 12: survival analysis. Critical Care. 2004;8:389–394. DOI: 10.1186/ cc2955

[145] Wen W, Ding J, Sun W, Fu J, Chen Y, Wu K, Ning B, Han T, Huang L, Chen C, Xie D, Li Z, Feng G, Wu M, Xie W, Wang H. Cyclin G1-mediated epithelial-mesenchymal transition via phosphoinositide 3-kinase/Akt signaling facilitates liver cancer progression. Hepatology. 2012;55:1787–1798. DOI: 10.1002/hep.25596

[146] Loret N, Denys H, Tummers P, Berx G. The role of epithelial-to-mesenchymal plasticity in ovarian cancer progression and therapy resistance. Cancers. 2019;11:6. DOI: 10.3390/cancers11060838.

[147] Pashai N, Hao H, All A, Gupta S, Chaerkady R, De Los Angeles A,

Gearhart JD, Kerr CL. Genome-wide profiling of pluripotent cells reveals a unique molecular signature of human embryonic germ cells. PLoS One. 2012;7: 6. DOI: 10.1371/journal.pone.0039088.

[148] Lehne G, Grasmo-Wendler UH, Berner JM, Meza-Zepeda LA, Adamsen BL, Flack A, Reiner A, Clausen OP, Hovig E, Myklebost O. Upregulation of stem cell genes in multidrug resistant K562 leukemia cells. Leukemia Research. 2009; 33: 1379–1385. DOI: 10.1016/j.leukres.2009.03.028

[149] Xiao AW, Jia Y, Baughn LB, Pearce KE, Pitel BA, Aster JC, Dal Cin P, Xiao S. IGH rearrangement in myeloid neoplasms. Haematologica. 2020;105: e315–e317. DOI: 10.3324/haematol.2020.246744

[150] Gordon EM, Szeto C, Ravicz JR, Reddy S, Morse M, Chawla S, Hall FL. Abstract 2556: Enhanced expression of human cyclin G1 (CCNG1) gene in metastatic cancer, a novel biomarker in development for CCNG1 inhibitor therapy. Cancer Research. 2019;79:2556–2556. DOI: 10.1158/1538-7445. AM2019-2556

[151] Singh A, Settleman J. EMT, cancer stem cells and drug resistance: an emerging axis of evil in the war on cancer. Oncogene. 2010;29:4741–4751. DOI: 10.1038/onc.2010.215

[152] Bandopadhyay M, Sarkar N, Datta S, Das D, Pal A, Panigrahi R, Banerjee A, Panda CK, Das C, Chakrabarti S, Chakravarty R. Hepatitis B virus X protein mediated suppression of miRNA-122 expression enhances hepatoblastoma cell proliferation through cyclin G1-p53 axis. Infectious Agents and Cancer. 2016;11:40. DOI: 10.1186/s13027-016-0085-6.

[153] Desai N, Trieu V, Damascelli B, Soon-Shiong P. SPARC expression correlates with tumor response to albumin-bound paclitaxel in head and neck cancer patients. Translational Oncology. 2009;2:59–64. DOI: 10.1593/tlo.09109

[154] Schneeweiss A, Seitz J, Smetanay K, Schuetz F, Jaeger D, Bachinger A, Zorn M, Sinn HP, Marmé F. Efficacy of nab-paclitaxel does not seem to be associated with SPARC expression in metastatic breast cancer. Anticancer Research. 2014;34: 6609–6616.

[155] Neesse A, Frese KK, Chan DS, Bapiro TE, Howat WJ, Richards FM, Ellenrieder V, Jodrell DI, Tuveson DA. SPARC independent drug delivery and antitumour effects of nab-paclitaxel in genetically engineered mice. Gut. 2014; 63:974–983. DOI: 10.1136/gutjnl-2013-305559

[156] Hidalgo M, Plaza C, Musteanu M, Illei P, Brachmann CB, Heise C, Pierce D, Lopez-Casas PP, Menendez C, Tabernero J, Romano A, Wei X, Lopez-Rios F, Von Hoff DD. SPARC expression did not predict efficacy of nab-paclitaxel plus gemcitabine or gemcitabine alone for metastatic pancreatic cancer in an exploratory analysis of the phase III MPACT trial. Clinical Cancer Research. 2015;21:4811–4818. DOI: 10.1158/1078-0432.CCR-14-3222

[157] Rugo HS, Barry WT, Moreno-Aspitia A, Lyss AP, Cirricione C, Leung E, Mayer EL, Naughton M, Toppmeyer D, Carey LA, Perez EA, Hudis C, Winer EP. Randomized phase III trial of paclitaxel once per week compared with nanoparticle albumin-bound nab-paclitaxel once per week or ixabepilone with bevacizumab ss first-line chemotherapy for locally recurrent or metastatic breast cancer: CALGB 40502/NCCTG N063H (Alliance). Journal of Clinical Oncology. 2015;33:2361–2369. DOI: 10.1200/JCO.2014.59.5298

[158] Huang TT, Parab S, Burnett R, Diago O, Ostertag D, Hofman FM,

Espinoza FL, Martin B, Ibañez CE, Kasahara N, Gruber HE, Pertschuk D, Jolly DJ, Robbins JM. Intravenous administration of retroviral replicating vector, Toca 511, demonstrates therapeutic efficacy in orthotopic immune-competent mouse glioma model. Human Gene Therapy. 2015;26: 82–93. DOI: 10.1089/hum.2014.100

[159] Hiraoka K, Inagaki A, Kato Y, Huang TT, Mitchell LA, Kamijima S, Takahashi M, Matsumoto H, Hacke K, Kruse CA, Ostertag D, Robbins JM, Gruber HE, Jolly DJ, Kasahara N. Retroviral replicating vector–mediated gene therapy achieves long-term control of tumor recurrence and leads to durable anticancer immunity. Neuro-Oncology. 2017;19:918–929. DOI: 10.1093/neuonc/nox038

[160] Hossain JA, Marchini A, Fehse B, Bjerkvig R, Miletic H. Suicide gene therapy for the treatment of high-grade glioma: past lessons, present trends, and future prospects. Neuro-Oncology Advances. 2020;2:vdaa013. DOI: 10.1093/noajnl/vdaa013

[161] MedCity News. Tocagen Phase III Study in Brain Cancer Fails, Sending Shares Plummeting [Internet]. 2019. Available from: https://medcitynews. com/2019/09/tocagen-phase-iii-study-in-brain-cancer-fails-sending-shares-plummeting [Accessed: 2020-11-23]

[162] Rahman M, Sawyer WG, Lindhorst S, Deleyrolle LP, Harrison JK, Karachi A, Dastmalchi F, Flores-Toro J, Mitchell DA, Lim M, Gilbert MR, Reardon DA. Adult immuno-oncology: using past failures to inform the future. Neuro-Oncology. 2020;22:1249–1261. DOI: 10.1093/neuonc/noaa116

[163] Miller K, Abraham JH, Rhodes L, Roberts R. Use of the word "cure" in oncology. Journal of Oncology Practice. 2013;9:e136–e140. DOI: 10.1200/ JOP.2012.000806

[164] Tralongo P, Maso LD, Surbone A, Santoro A, Tirelli U, Sacchini V, Pinto C, Crispino S, Ferraù F, Mandoliti G, Tonini G, Russo A, Santini D, Madeddu A, Panebianco V, Pergolizzi S, Respini D, Rolfo C, Bongiovanni M, De Lorenzo F, Spatola C, Di Raimondo F, Terenziani M, Peeters M, Castoro C. Use of the word "cured" for cancer patients —implications for patients and physicians: the Siracusa charter. Current Oncology. 2015;22:e38–e40. DOI: 10.3747/co.22.2287

[165] Aguilera-Rojas M, Sharbati S, Stein T, Einspanier R. Deregulation of miR-27a may contribute to canine fibroblast activation after coculture with a mast cell tumour cell line. FEBS Open Bio. 2020;10:802–816. DOI: 10.1002/ 2211-5463.12831

[166] ClinicalTrials. Expanded Access for DeltaRex-G for Advanced Pancreatic Cancer and Sarcoma [Internet]. 2020. Available from: https://clinicaltrials.g ov/ct2/show/NCT04091295 [Accessed: 2020-11-22]

www.ingramcontent.com/pod-product-compliance
Lightning Source LLC
Chambersburg PA
CBHW081246190326
41458CB00016B/5935